BRIAN CLEMENT
C.N, N.M.D., Ph.D.
Director, The Hippocrates Health Institute

LONGEVITY:
ENJOYING LONG LIFE
WITHOUT LIMITS

Preface by Jacques-Pascal Cusin

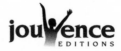

jouvence
EDITIONS

The information in this volume is not intended as a substitute for consultation
with healthcare professionals. Each individual's health concerns should be
evaluated by a qualified professional.

Printed in France

ISBN 13: 978-0-9759037-0-4
ISBN 10: 0-9759037-0-5

TABLE OF CONTENTS

A SECOND OPINION

Dear Readers: Please note that this book constitutes the accumulation and compilation of the learning, experience and understanding of the author and of The Hippocrates Health Institute — which over its more than half-century of research and application has made it possible for many thousands of people to maximize their health and find fulfillment.

In conjunction with the philosophy of The Hippocrates Health Institute and the author as stated herein and expressed in this book, all readers have absolute authority over their diets, health and functioning. Therefore, The Hippocrates Health Institute, the contents of this book, and the author are neither intended to nor in any way replace the absolute self- determination of each reader.

Readers are free to use the information in their own way at their own pace, while utilizing, whenever necessary, the counsel of qualified, experienced, appropriate practitioners, doctors, and/or other medical professionals with full knowledge and application of the following self referential considerations: Age; gender; level of health; health problems; physical, emotional, psychological, situational, logistical status and/or limitations/impairments thereto; relevant circumstances (i.e., health problems, genetic history, familial situation, occupation, domicile, local and global environment, pregnancy, menopause, availability of recommended foods, etc.); level of fitness; and all other relevant considerations.

Everyone who uses this book — for self or others — must consider and implement the following conditions:

A. The individual — not any entity outside the individual, whether a family member, friend, practitioner, pundit, group, book, or system — is the source and continuity of all health, healing and self maintenance. Therefore, this book — like all other external sources of information — is merely an adjunct to each individual's absolute autonomy over his/her life and health.

B. Every individual is unique. Therefore, before the application of any mode of procedure to any individual, all the following facts and factors about that individual must be considered and applied: Gender, age and genetic history; current

health and health history (physical, psychological and emotional) and any impairment thereto; physical condition, level of exercise and other activities and diet; particular circumstances as pregnancy and puberty; climate, season and geographical location; schedule and occupation, as well as any and all other individual and general relevant conditions, circumstances and considerations.

C. No matter how beneficial, no mode of procedure can be useful unless it is utilized properly, both in individual instances and with the required regularity; and all modes benefit from the input of qualified, excellent practitioners.

ACKNOWLEDGEMENTS

Let me gratefully acknowledge the many meaningful contributions to this work by people of every age, sex, race, place and profession. Because these contributors love, respect and appreciate life, they are living representatives of the principles in this book.

Every day — every moment — is precious. We must honor this by living life to its fullest, not only for ourselves but for others. Celebrate every exhilarating second; travel paths that lead you to the best and most positive ways of everyday living.

Let me express my profound appreciation and gratitude to my friend, George Kovacs, Ph.D., Communications Consultant to The Hippocrates Health Institute. Without his comprehensive and unrestrained dedication, knowledge, professionalism and contributions this volume would not exist.

My children — Daly, Danielle, Gail, and Blake — are endless sources of love and learning. This book is dedicated to them and to my beloved wife, Anna Maria. When I met my best friend and lifelong companion, Anna Maria Gahns, on a sunny April day in Stockholm, I knew immediately that I had reached the fulfillment that would make it possible for me to serve not only my immediate family but my human and worldwide families as well.

FOREWORD

A radiant and long life is within the reach of all. The Longevity Program's core concept demonstrates and validates fifty years of research and application in life extension conducted at the renowned Hippocrates Health Institute. Increasing life expectancy in the western world can greatly impact health concerns and their economic fallout, social order and its emotional components and ultimately can dramatically and positively improve the economy of the world. By shepherding your body and mind your ability to become a contributing member of society is significantly enhanced. This lifesaving act also benefits your family, friends, countrymen and humanity as a whole. The human toll and economic havoc that illness brings can be silenced by adopting a responsible lifestyle.

Your physical body is constantly exposed to oxidization, a phenomenon that mimics storms attacking land. Your body, in the same way, is the recipient of devastation when free radicals erode the very anatomy that houses you. This ongoing war is precipitated by breathing polluted air and water, consuming chemically laden and processed foods, and an out of control mind that allows stress to govern its every action. Together with the abundant fear that reigns over us, this lethal concoction sparks premature aging and death.

Dr. Brian Clement and a few other visionaries believe our contemporary world has dramatically changed and it is time to go back to our roots. Clement speaks out about the problems we face, but at the same moment, gives you concrete resolutions to resolve them. Not only can we alleviate the physical and emotional ravages that result in disorder and disease, but we can raise ourselves above them achieving a level of energy, vitality and authenticity that brings inevitable joy. Dr. Clement's message is simple: Utilize living thoughts, living exercise, living relationships (including sexual) and living food. When you have the self respect and confidence to do so, you will achieve balance in the process of maturing.

There is a new anti-aging science that spotlights the importance of proper lifestyle in the conquest of silencing disease and premature death. Relaxation, rest and sleep are equally important in living vitally. In fact, Clement thinks that anti-aging conjures up an impossible dream and would rather look at it as either the "medicine to increase time" or "active aging." The ultimate purpose for all of these efforts is to do our best to make our own life and the lives of others more fruitful. This global movement began at the Hippocrates Health Institute over half a century ago when its mission of making every man, woman and child on the earth as healthy and happy as possible ignited. The beauty that is derived from this simple, yet profound process is that of "youthifying." Youth's appeal is a result of good physical, emotional, mental and spiritual practice. The burden of unhealthy aging is realized when we allow these resources to dwindle and erode through bad habits. A fresh and exciting voyage will begin when you surrender your limitations and utilize your imagination.

Brian Clement suggests that we give special attention to our brain's health since it is the epicenter of everything. When we permit this vital organ to weaken, the result is confusion, chaos and stagnation. The current upsurge of memory disorders or so called neuro-degenerative disease stems from our disconnection with the nourishment, calisthenics and purification of the mind. The first step in life extension is to pay critical attention to your head. This book is not only educational but is a practical tool that you can use from now until you are 150! All of you who choose to allow time to flow the way that nature wants it, will flourish in frequenting the viable lifestyle choices that are offered in this Longevity Program. When you do what is right, you will add years to your life.

Jacques-Pascal Cusin
Health and food consultant
Nutri-therapist
Author

INTRODUCTION

Longevity is not merely an idea; it is an absolute reality for those who choose to be responsible for their lives and their world. Now in my fourth decade of helping people live better longer, I initiated, developed and expanded The Longevity Program — a viable system for the unlimited reservoir of vitality that marks a thriving long life and an abundance of happiness. This internationally renowned system of daily success promotes your potential and liberates your potency.

Graceful aging is our natural birthright; only by living unnaturally do we deny it to ourselves and others. Unnatural living generates unhappiness, lack of fulfillment, resentment and bitterness, all of which imprint their negative marks on us as we progress through life. It is inevitable, then, that we suffer through life, struggle as we age, and then die too young. This process can be altered only by the one who confronts it — you. And you can change it only by making natural, life affirming, positive choices.

It is pointless to blame anyone or anything outside yourself for your degeneration. No predestination — including genetics — can trap you into patterns that you neither create nor sustain. Because this is so, you can undo or terminate these patterns.

So let us look forward to your glorious and positive longevity. The quality of your life is determined by the quality of your choices. First, you choose to think positively. Then you act in a way that is consistent with those affirmative thoughts. Finally, you fuel yourself and create newly broadened horizons with the bountiful banquet of vegetarian offerings. These foods, so full of life, give you strength, vigor and unlimited mental and physical potential. Your newly invigorated self celebrates a regenerated anatomy and a spirit that flows through time with ageless energy.

Renewed, you are inspired to embrace life harmoniously. Your passion will inspire your purpose, invigorate your activities and illuminate your horizons. This book is your guide to an enriching longevity, with a step-by-step program to help you rebuild your life on nature's solid foundations, freeing you to concentrate on your fascinating future.

CHAPTER ONE

THE HISTORY OF AGING

Our bodies constantly regenerate themselves. As developed cells complete their tasks, they are replaced by healthy new cells often created in our bone marrow. While we have always known that we age, we have always questioned why it happens anatomically. The mistaken notion was that the Fountain of Youth was outside our bodies; many people spent their lives searching for it. The secret has always been that the possibility of constant renewal exists within each of us.

Living life fully and positively guarantees enduring health and happiness. Self-respect fuels a healthy longevity and creates respect for all life. This respect is not abstract; indeed, it is extremely practical, manifested by passionate creativity and positive, life serving goals. We can actually elevate our thought processes, diet, exercise, rest and interactions to ennoble ourselves.

At the beginnings of human life, we lived far longer, on average, than we do in this supposedly advanced modern era. Why? The answer is simple: The farther back we go, the more we were in harmony with nature; the further ahead we moved in time, the more backward we became at natural living. So to return to longevity, we must return to nature, return nature to itself, and return ourselves to our natural selves.

Historical data indicate that many people in all parts of the world have lived long and actively fulfilling lives. Today that is a rarity, despite the claims of certain pseudo-scientists who falsely maintain that we are living longer than our ancestors did. In the past, infectious diseases such as plagues and other water-borne invaders were responsible for most premature deaths worldwide.

Comparative statistics of recent generations indicate that life expectancy was approximately twenty years less for our great-grandparents than it is for us. Unfortunately, some "scientists" manufacture these statistics without considering the impact of infant mortality, even though techno-logical medical advances have significantly diminished the incidence of such deaths. Contagious diseases, at least in the Western Hemisphere, are now under better control, but until medical technology was developed and modern diagnostic technology blossomed, approximately 25 percent of children died at birth or in infancy. So, if some people live beyond 100 but many die in infancy, the average life expectancy is approximately 50. By overlooking past infant mortality figures, we dramatically increase the statistical age in our time to the mid-70s, while in fact we are not living longer but are being deceived into believing so — all while we are under more stress than ever.

The disease rate of people living in cultures more attuned to nature has always been low and their life expectancy has always been high. Living in harmony with nature has always been — and will always be — the only way to enjoy a long, full, fulfilling life. Eating appropriate quantities of organic living foods, doing satisfying work, enjoying healthy exercise, maintaining positive relationships, and nurturing constructive thoughts constitute the support system of energized life extension.

Historically, most societies have demonstrated profound respect for those who achieved maturity. Today, that honor is inappropriately denied to those who have earned it; instead, the mere chronological happen-stance of youth is glorified. The psychological impact of this lack of regard is twofold: Once, children wanted to mature quickly in order to generate esteem. Now, today's youth — and many adults — want to remain young forever. This stigma against aging has provoked not only the scourge of ageism but also many false, unnecessary and harmful sys-tems to combat natural aging.

Many of us wrongly believe that aging involves cumulative degenera-tion of the body and the will, as well as indecisiveness, loss of memory and mental capacity, and relentlessly degenerating health and sexual vital-ity. However, if you live a responsible life, you can navigate your maturi-ty through calm, supportive and productive seas. For more than half a century, The Hippocrates Health Institute has been the vessel for thousands of rejuvenated elders, transporting them toward their best years. When you take charge of your life, it becomes possible to enjoy a productive aging experience instead of one that is counterproductive.

CHAPTER TWO

MODERN AGING: ATTITUDE IS EVERYTHING

Many of our parents and grandparents were prematurely exhausted by the demands of life; their concern about early degeneration and demise contributed to that process. Leisure time was rare, work was draining, families were large, homes were humble and crowded, and household tasks were demanding and endless. Such self-destructive habits as smoking, alcohol consumption, increasingly bad diets and restrictive thinking caused us to age fast and die young, and a peculiarly misplaced sense of trust left people vulnerable, leading them to believe that external forces would sustain and save them.

In many ways, our recent ancestors were a curious combination of naïve, prematurely ancient and childlike; modern high-speed living causes us to degenerate even more quickly. But instead of exhausting ourselves with activity, we destroy ourselves by the consequences of our activity: pollution, destructive diets, large-scale destruction and the way we distance ourselves from vital living. Catastrophic epidemics are annihilating us, and like willful children hurtling into harm's way we rush headlong toward our own destruction.

We must stop this self-destructive cycle. We must instead become informed adults who aspire to, and work toward, long, fruitful, healthy lives. To accomplish this, we need to clarify our thinking, elevate our awareness, and energize our spirit; this positive activity keeps the body vital and the self vibrant.

Visualize yourself in your mature years: You awaken from a refreshing sleep; you are full of enthusiasm, energy and elation. You fill your day, including your diet and exercise, with rewarding activity, mutually beneficial relationships and healthy interaction with nature.

Youth is eternal, because it begins with *you*. Age does not determine how you function: *You* do. In fact, maturity offers you the best of both worlds: Continuity of youthful vitality combined with a mature appreciation of it.

Rueful recollections of youth impede the appreciation of maturity: Do not look back. Instead, appreciate today and anticipate tomorrow. With every step forward, you develop vitality and increase passion. Remember the wise insights of our respected elders, baseball's Leroy "Satchel" Paige, and Don Quixote in *Man of La Mancha*. Paige said, "Don't look back; something might be gaining on you." Don Quixote said, "Look always forward; in last year's nest, there are no birds this year."

A continued romance with life yields a banquet of rewards and a mutually successful relationship: If you love life, it will love you back. The harmony between you and life will expand to include you and the entire world. Your heightened perception and intensified living will reward you with unlimited potential and life as a vibrant, vital participant.

A 106-year-old Asian visitor once courteously interrupted a Hippocrates seminar by telling us that when he was 80 he had read one of our books about nutrition and had thrived thereafter by living solely on a bio-organic diet. It had been his dream that someday he would cross the ocean and visit the Institute. One of the seminar participants asked him to reveal the secret of his longevity. He smiled and said, "Every day, when I awaken, I thank God for everything that I have; and then I find a way to give something back. Doing this removes the burden of carrying unnecessary and unwanted baggage."

Most of us are merely what we accumulate; however, a fulfilling longevity requires the elimination of excess. A light, nourishing diet, positive thought, exhilarating exercise, spiritual purpose and a daily commitment to living with integrity are cornerstones of the long and fruitful life.

CHAPTER THREE

ACTIVE MIND, AGILE BRAIN, AGING THOUGHTFULLY

Neuronal connections circulate throughout the body from our extremities to our internal organs. There are, literally, many miles of nerve fibers in each human body, all of which eventually connect to the brain.

The most important ally in improvement and maintenance of mental, physical, emotional and spiritual health is our continuing exploration and liberation of the brain and its multi-faceted existence and potential. Independent studies at both the Max Planck Institute in Heidelberg, Germany, and at Vanderbilt University in Nashville, Tennessee, have proven the powerful potential of a single brain cell. These studies have proven that activating just one cell in the brain results in spontaneous movement. This knowledge will eventually benefit not only those whose movements are hampered but those who are otherwise impaired or suffering no impairment whatever.

The brain's unlimited ultimate capacity clearly indicates that, as astonishing as our brains have been so far, their potential is immeasurable. It is the responsibility of each individual to magnify that potential, because the brain is the governing center of each person's physical, mental, emotional and spiritual universe. As Marguerite Holloway has written in a special issue of *Scientific American* devoted to the brain, "Score one for believers in the adage, 'Use it or lose it.' Targeted mental and physical exercise seem to improve the brain in unexpected ways."

In *Brain Longevity*, Dr. Dharma Singh Khalsa says that we have the ability to prevent the hormones cortisol and adrenaline from causing our brain to age prematurely. Diet, exercise, meditation, prayer, proper rest and sleep and legitimate supplementation are the required elements that help to sustain and maximize the vitality and functioning of the brain.

The brain is the unifying physical component, guardian and generator of the four aspects of life: Body, mind, emotion and spirit. Therefore, only by refining the brain can we enlarge our own lives and all of life. So be refined: Use your mind!

One of the benefits of maturity is the accumulated wisdom gathered in the brain and utilized by the mind. *Time* magazine's special-issue cover story, "How to Live to Be 100," provides critical insight into the important connection between sustained brain activity and a long, rewarding life. For this feature, centenarians (humans aged 100 or more) were interviewed; they uniformly agreed that an agile mind promotes active, productive, gratifying longevity. Dedication, perseverance, focus, a positive attitude and endurance are fundamental ingredients that coordinate the development of wisdom with the advancement of maturity.

Most "longevians" — our word for people who live long lives — have one of two diametrically divergent attitudes: They are either extremely positive or irritatingly disagreeable. How can we explain the fact that two such opposite philosophies can sustain equal longevity? The answer may be that both procedures keep the neurons of the brain active, energetic and vital.

Many brilliant intellectuals have continued to make remarkable contributions well into their maturity; philosopher Bertrand Russell, author George Bernard Shaw, producer George Abbott, actors Charlie Chaplin and Jean-Pierre Aumont, artists Michelangelo, Grandma Moses and Willem de Kooning, playwright, Arthur Miller, humanitarian and founder of The Hippocrates Health Institute Ann Wigmore, and many others throughout the world.

EXERCISES
TO KEEP YOUR BRAIN VITAL

You can keep your brain agile and your thought processes fertile in many fascinating ways.

Canadian researcher Dr. Danielle Laurin has conducted studies exploring the relationship between insufficient physical activity and the risk of cognitive impairment, a serious risk that may cause dementia, senility and Alzheimer's disease. She and her associates generated research based on a random sampling of 9,008 men and women over the age of 65; among the 6,434 people who were deemed cognitively functional for the purposes of the study, 4,615 fulfilled the entire five-year requirement of that study. The results revealed that 3,894 of the participants remained free of cognitive impairment, 436 were diagnosed as having some mild cognitive impairment but no dementia, and 285 were diagnosed with dementia.

The scientists concluded not only that exercise is beneficial for mental stability, but that more intense and regular exercise benefits brain functions and thought processes more intensely and profoundly, and for longer periods of time. The results of this published study include the benefits of mild to moderate exercise for people over the age of 40:

A. protects brain cells from toxins, including free radicals and excess glutamate;

B. repairs DNA to protect the brain — and the rest of the body — against programmed cell death;

C. reduces the risk — by half — of cognitive impairment and other dementia caused by Attention Deficit Disorder (ADD) and other such impairments among those 65 and older;

D. preserves the complete mental functioning of those past 70;

E. reduces the risk of heart disease and stroke by modifying cholesterol levels and improving the metabolizing of fats;

F. improves the delivery of oxygen, glucose and blood to the tissues of the brain and the rest of the body;

G. diminishes the risk of diabetes by facilitating the balancing effect of insulin in blood sugar (glucose) while increasing the ratio of lean to fat mass in the body;

H. minimizes osteoporosis and other bone-degenerating problems when combined with resistance exercise;

I. combats lethargy, depression and melancholia;

J. reduces the incidence of colon cancer, breast cancer, and other cancers and infirmities;

K. reduces the age-related problem of falling by improving muscle tone, endurance and balance, which also reduces the likelihood and intensity of strokes.

My own work with many tens of thousands of people has led me to understand the importance of ten essential activities to stimulate the neurons of the brain in order to increase clarity and vitality of thought and invigorate for intellectual challenges:

1. GOALS: When you awaken, write three objectives to accomplish that day, listed in order of priority. Then, as you fulfill each, write how you have done so.

2. INSIGHTS: Make each day a resource for discovering literature that stimulates positive thought, including not only books but distinguished periodicals and unique volumes among your choices.

3. INSOUNDS: Similarly, listen each day to sounds that soothe, stimulate and strengthen mind and spirit — classical music, opera, jazz, rock, musical theater and more.

4. NATURE: Immerse yourself in the sights, sounds and sensations of nature. One of the many benefits of longevity is continued harmonious merging with the natural world with which we are inextricably intertwined.

5. INTERACTION: We are part not only of nature but also of all of life; therefore, we must interact in mutually beneficial ways with other people who share our world. Harmonious interaction with others elevates you, them and the world that we all share.

6. VISUAL ART (COLOR THERAPY): Once you have seen the beauty of nature and other life, seek its representation in the great visual art that rewards us with textures, sensations, associations and revelations. Nature provides the vibrant colors, glorious configurations, and imposing images that excite the brain and intensify creativity.

7. DRAMATIC ARTS —THEATER AND MOVING PICTURES: Drama is among our oldest, most respected, and fascinating arts. It stimulates the senses, increases our understanding, elevates our humanity, engages our essence, and entertains us. However, as with all human undertakings, the performing arts offer us a range of options from fulfilling to frustrating. One of the many benefits of progressive maturity is the wisdom-acquired ability to select those plays and films and TV shows that inspire and ennoble us.

8. CONTEMPLATION (MEDITATION/PRAYER): Contemplation is one of those rare activities that both invigorates and calms at the same time. This means that you are both vibrant and at rest during and after meditation. As this stimulates the brain, it also stimulates every aspect of the self: Mental, physical, emotional and spiritual. Continued implementation of formal meditative techniques benefits and builds longevity.

9. CHI QUING and TAI CHI: These Asian traditions, established to promote the life force that is within each of us, unify and coordinate mind, body and spirit, creating the internal harmony that facilitates focus and precision.

10. FULFILLMENT: Achieving positive goals yields a fulfillment that satisfies our core. This rewarding process activates the cells of the brain (neurons) and creates an abundance of endorphins, chemistries that inspire confidence, security and tranquility. Poet Robert Browning illustrated the connection between this fulfillment and triumphant longevity in his poem, "Rabbi Ben Ezra," which begins:

> *"Grow old along with me!*
> *The best is yet to be,*
> *The last of life for which the first was made . . ."*

RELAX AND SMILE:
THINK WELL TO LIVE WELL

In his book *Old Age Is Not for Sissies*, TV personality Art Linkletter writes that the word "attitude" might be the most important in any language, because our attitude indicates how we are at every age, making some wither before their time and others blossom in their prime. Actress Betty White (whose own career illustrates formidable longevity) has said that intellectual vigor sustains vitality irrespective of age.

In *Arnott's Guide to Turning Back the Clock*, Dr. Robert Arnott suggests that legitimate athletic competition at maturity is as beneficial as it is during early development. The benefit of mature athletics is that the focus shifts from beating the opponent to sustaining the participant. This philosophy is in accord with Linkletter's; both men maintain that positive attitude is the foundation of productive activity at every age.

Jeanne Marceau, a guest at The Institute, told me when she was 97 that she continues to discover refreshing aspects in herself, others and nature every day.

Limitation is a fabrication of inhibition; free your mind and you free yourself. The resulting freedom allows you to fulfill your dreams and then dream newer, bolder, grander ones. And, of course, each of us must choose and maintain the best direction for ourselves without intruding on anyone else — that way, we can all relax and smile.

FUEL THE BRAIN PROPERLY
BY FEEDING THE BRAIN PROPERLY

Although there is much discussion (and availability) of nutrients for the body, it is amazing how seldom nutrition designed exclusively for the brain is discussed or offered. In truth, there are many fine nutritional contributions for the brain, and these offerings benefit other parts of the body as well. Here is a list of some of these brain-benefiting sources:

ALPHA-LIPOIC ACID: This small but powerful molecule enters the brain to protect it from free radical damage. Alpha-lipoic acid activates glutathione — the most powerful antioxidant in our cells — which stimulates the ability of each to absorb free radicals, thereby neutralizing their negative effects. Since international research has revealed that free radicals attack brain cells (neurons), the use of alpha-lipoic acid prevents or limits the damage caused by these free radicals. Studies also indicate that this powerful preventive agent helps remove lead from brain tissue.

BRAIN ALGAE: Sublingual (under the tongue) use of these algae extracts protects the entire brain while reestablishing healthy channels of neuronal activity. The 50-percent protein content of blue-green algae helps alleviate depression by reinvigorating those parts of the brain in which it appears.

B VITAMINS: Our use of B vitamins that are derived exclusively from whole foods benefits the nervous system and helps the brain create and sustain the neurotransmitters that embody thoughts and moods. Members of the B vitamin family are essential for sustained energy, balanced hormones, and healthy mental and cardiovascular functioning. Research indicates that deficiencies of B vitamins cause lethargy, depression, dementia and nerve degeneration.

CAT'S CLAW (UNA DA GATO) The essence of this South American plant helps counteract and/or prevent Attention Deficit Disorder (ADD), which attacks not only children but also those adults who are facing or have dementia.

COENZYME (CoQ10): This essential enzyme lives inside the mitochondria of our cells; it helps to convert oxygen into the usable energy called adenosine triphate. CoQ10 protects cells — including neurons — from mutating into potential physical and mental problems, including memory loss, dementia, senility and Alzheimer's disease. Research indicates that this antioxidant inhibits the development of brain dysfunctions by almost 50 percent.

DHEA (DEHYDROEPIANDROSTERONE SULFATE): This beneficial steroid derived from wild yam extract is useful in the production of estrogen and testosterone. It also helps prevent the deterioration and loss of brain cells.

HEMP (OMEGA OILS): Hemp seeds are plentiful, efficient sources of the oils Omega-3 and Omega-6. Germination of these tiny seeds turns them into usable fatty acids. Their easy access to the ventricles of the brain barrier helps nourish and rebuild the structure of the brain.

KAVA KAVA: A beneficial herbal extract used throughout the world to combat melancholia, which it does by reinvigorating the brain-cell mechanisms that stagnate when one is depressed.

MELATONIN: Periodic use of this helpful hormone counteracts the disturbances and deprivation of sleep that are associated with unhealthy aging. My clinical research indicates that daily long-term use of melatonin disrupts the enzyme functioning of the liver and gallbladder, so it must be used for brief periods with long intervals of non-use between each period. Its use must also be supervised by a competent, sympathetic health practitioner.

NONI: This South Pacific fruit possesses unique chemistries that activate and regenerate the receptor points of our cells, directly promoting the life and functioning of those cells. Noni helps stall and control the potential degeneration of the brain, as well as providing many other benefits to the entire body.

OXYGEN (SUPPLEMENTAL): Many excellent and effective forms of supplemental oxygen are available that nourish, activate and intensify brain function.

PHYCOMIN: This unique extract of blue-green algae, imbued with phytochemicals, combats patterns of counterproductive brain chemistry. It has been of great benefit in my work, serving to counteract various depressive disorders.

RUTIN: This member of the B vitamin family stimulates and intensifies healthy circulatory activity, thereby strengthening and stabilizing the functioning and balance of veins, capillaries and related systems.

SEA WATER: Because the chemical composition of pristine sea water is similar to that of our blood, drinking that water nourishes, reinvigorates and replenishes our very lifeblood.

VITAMIN C and VITAMIN E: Consumed in its whole-food supplemental form, this combination of Vitamin C and Vitamin E provides many benefits, including reduction and elimination of Attention Deficit Disorder (ADD), protection of brain cells (neurons) from the formation of free radicals, and control and repression of infections. This potent combination is also a natural anticoagulant, facilitating unrestricted blood flow.

Proper use of these supplements — and many others — helps to preserve and enhance the functioning of the entire body, including the brain. These nutriceuticals expedite the maintenance and reconstruction of the entire brain and of its constituent 10 trillion individual cells.

NOTE: *All herbs and nutritional supplements should be taken in their living whole-food forms to assure the proper and complete beneficial effects of their subcultures and co-factors. Taking isolated nutrients is counterproductive to health; as a service to robust longevity, always use these building blocks of vitality in their complete form.*

CHAPTER FOUR

NUTRITION:
FEED YOUR BRAIN
AND FUEL YOUR BODY

We need a healthy brain to understand that we must feed the brain to keep it healthy. In other words, we must sustain the brain in two ways — by constant use and consistent nourishment, because we need a perceptive brain to comprehend how amazing the brain is. It has been said that most people have more than 6,000 thoughts each day, and that most of these thoughts are regularly recycled and reconfigured according to their importance to our daily interactions. Every thought has some effect, no matter how subtle, on the brain, the body, other life, and the environment.

The remarkable brain consists of 85 trillion cells, of which 100 billion are neurons that constitute a connective network involving clusters of thousands of neurons. Although historically it had been believed that brain-related neurons and neuron functioning were exclusive to the brain, science has since demonstrated that neurons in other parts of the body are equally critical to brain chemistry, mental functioning, and thought processes. The digestive system and elimination canal produce two-thirds of the body's serotonin, the chemical that transmits neurons to create and sustain happiness. These chemistries, along with other neurons and natural chemistries, flow throughout the intestinal tract, also affecting the brain and its many important activities.

The brain and the stomach are in constant communication, so what you eat has a direct and immediate influence on what you think and how you feel — as well as *how* you think and *what* you feel. Consumption of bad "foods" produces negative feelings, self-destructive thoughts, conflict, impaired rest, disturbed sleep, even suicide. Good food results in good feelings, joyful thoughts, harmony, complete rest, fulfilling sleep and a positive attitude.

The brain is so complex that no similar structure exists in the rest of the body, the rest of nature or even the rest of the known universe. The closest parallel — remote at best — is the infinite drops of water in an ocean. Think of each drop as part of the infinitely complex interactive cell structure of the brain, flowing with ideas, fluid in its functioning and dominating the whole. The interactive junctures between and among neurons are called dendrites, and the gaps between the junctures are called synapses. It is across these electrically charged gaps that information travels.

A study conducted at Salpetr Hospital in Paris revealed that the brains and bodies of people who suffer from Alzheimer's disease contain 60 percent less selenium than the systems of those who are not impaired. Selenium promotes the production of dopamine, the brain chemical that enhances positive moods and promotes clarity of thought.

Messages in the brain travel like radio waves, so much so that the brain's communication system literally involves messenger cells, neurotransmitters (the messages themselves, consisting mostly of amino acids), and receptor cells. Individual proteins create and fuel individual neurotransmitters: For example, tryptophan creates serotonin, the neurotransmitter that conveys positive emotions such as happiness. Phenylalanine creates and sustains dopamine, which induces calm, and adrenaline, which generates motivation. These and other components are built and sustained by the essential fats (which, as part of the brain, become phospholipids) that are found in algae and sprouted seeds as well as the raw material of amino acids that is readily available from the protein found in a variety of vegetarian foods. The incontrovertible fact is that only vegetarian foods provide exceptional amounts of extraordinary proteins (amino acids).

Clearly, the maintenance and maximization of the brain require abundant protein, as well as vitamins, minerals and trace minerals. Each nutrient, individually and in combination, activates and facilitates the enzyme activity that induces, produces and promotes healthy, complete brain functioning and mental capacity.

The following five nutritional components produce and sustain optimal lifelong brain functioning:

ESSENTIAL FATS, PHOSPHOLIPIDS, AMINO ACIDS, GLUCOSE BALANCE and INTELLIGENCE-INDUCING NUTRIENTS

Let us discuss each individually:

ESSENTIAL FATS: These nutrients create and maintain the anatomical structure of the brain. Fatty acids provide your body — especially your brain — with substances called Omega-3 and Omega-6, Alpha-linolenic acid, EPA (eicosapentaenoic acid) and DHA (docosahexaenoic acid) are unsaturated, nutritious, healthy fats that are destroyed by cooking, heating and processing. Compared to people in the mid-19th century, unfortunately, most of today's population eats less than 17 percent of these necessary fats.

Omega-3 is critical to brain function for two reasons: It is part of the myelin, the essential anatomical structure of the brain, and it provides the materials from which the brain/body creates prostaglandins, the extremely active hormone-like substances that relax blood vessels (reducing blood pressure), maintain water balance, stimulate immunity, decrease inflammation and pain, and assist in the functioning of insulin in balancing blood sugar.

Prostaglandins regulate the functioning of neurotransmitters in the brain, and a chronic insufficiency of them causes depression, schizophrenia, behavioral problems, ADD, malaise, and suicidal inclinations.

Consuming Omega-3 in combination with animal-based products does not provide enough nutrition, because the saturated fats of animal fare interfere with the absorption of the healthy essential fatty acids that contain Omega-3. At Hammersmith Hospital in London, researchers have discovered that babies of breast-feeding vegan mothers have larger brains, superior mental capacity and greater intellectual potential than children of either omnivores or dairy-consuming vegetarians. Dr. Louise Thomas, one of the scientists involved in this study, believes that the balance of saturated fats as opposed to the imbalance of polyunsaturated fats in a person's fat tissue might be an indication of intelligence level. In another study that supports this contention, Dr. Donald Rudin of the University of California has proven that consumption of flax regulates and balances the functioning of schizophrenics and juvenile delinquents.

Omega-6 constitutes the other family of essential fatty acids. Although Omega-6 fats (linoleic acid) are necessary to the entire body, they are most prevalent in the brain. Linoleic acid is converted by the body into GLA (gamma linoleic acid), which creates and maintains the volume and mass of the anatomy of the brain.

Many of us attempt to avoid the necessary nutrient called fat. This is counterproductive, although it is wise to avoid the saturated fats that are plentiful in dairy products, meat, almost all processed and fried foods and even some margarines.

However, the essential fats that are plentiful in healthy raw vegan food are necessary to health; they are needed to build, maintain and heal the body and its various parts, including the brain. Most of us are almost devoid of these essential fats, and their absence causes learning difficulties, lack of concentration, impaired vision, dry and flaky scalp, soft and brittle nails, PMS and mammary tenderness, as well as dry, watery, itchy eyes, inflammatory arthritis, and elevated levels of blood pressure and blood lipids.

Worldwide, many women subject themselves to starvation diets, causing a chronic lack of healthy fats in their systems; as a result, the babies of these women are often born with the inadequately developed brains that cause Attention Deficit Disorder (ADD).

While avoiding all forms of saturated fats, you should make essential fatty acids approximately five percent of your diet. The best and most abundant sources of healthy fatty acids are to be found in The Longevity Diet.

YOUR BEST SOURCES OF ESSENTIAL FATS:

A. Sprouted sunflower, sprouted hemp, sprouted flax, sprouted sesame, sprouted almonds, sprouted pumpkin seeds and   sprouted garbanzo beans (chickpeas). The germinated forms of these seeds convert healthy fats into easy-to-digest fatty acids.

B. Sunflower green sprouts, pea green sprouts, fenugreek sprouts; each can be juiced to yield a pure nutritious liquid that contains significant amounts of healthy fatty acids.

C. Such hearty nuts as walnuts, macadamias and pecans contribute significantly to your supply and reserve of essential fatty acids.

D. The most complete sources of the essential fats of which the brain is composed are supplemental blue-green algae. Many of these algae are processed without being heated in order to extract concentrated levels of nutrients that can pass easily through the brain barrier in order to feed that brain.

E. Three other excellent brain foods are corn, borage and primrose oil, because they combat and minimize schizophrenia, limit the side effects of psychiatrically prescribed medications, and curtail bipolar disorder. After consumption, essential fats become phospholipids.

PHOSPHOLIPIDS: Phospholipids are the internal nutrients that literally create the energy in the brain that fosters and maintains its memory-generating and memory-retaining capabilities. These become more important as we mature and continue to accumulate memories.

YOUR BEST SOURCES OF SUBSTANCES THAT EVENTUALLY BECOME PHOSPHOLIPIDS:

In addition to the listed best sources of essential fats, phospholipids are also generated by sea vegetables, especially kelp, dulse, arame, wakame, tempeh (consumed in its raw form), and the various internationally available liquid forms of amino acids.

AMINO ACIDS: Proteins (amino acids) are the building blocks of the entire anatomy as well as of every cell and tissue of the body. They create and enhance the brain's internal network of communication. These body-converted proteins create and generate neurotransmission by creating and sustaining the neurotransmitters in the brain; amino acids constitute the substance of the messengers within the brain. Among the chemical neurotransmitters in the brain are the following:

1. Adrenaline, noradrenaline and dopamine: At proper levels, these active agents stimulate, motivate and activate   cognition as well as physical activity, assist in stress reduction and facilitate feelings of worth and happiness.

2. GABA generates post-stress relaxation and calms both brain and body.

3. Serotonin banishes the blues and encourages elation.

4. Acetylcholine improves memory, alertness and brain activity.

5. Tryptamines create harmonious universal metabolic rhythm and consistency.

AMINO ACIDS: An absence of amino acids from your diet encourages anxiety, depression, irritability, low blood pressure, impaired memory, improper development of hair and nail growth, indigestion, constant hunger, and lack of motivation, concentration and enthusiasm.

YOUR BEST SOURCES OF AMINO ACIDS:

Flower pollens, bee pollens, green algae, blue-green algae, wheatgrass juice, spelt juice, kamut juice, flaxseeds, sesame seeds, hemp seeds and mung bean sprouts.

GLUCOSE BALANCE: The most important nutrient for the brain and the nervous system is glucose: It is the fuel that gives the brain energy, just as petroleum fuels a vehicle. Our systems — including our brains — are solar-power once removed: We take the power of the sun as it is stored by plants in their absorption of hydrogen and oxygen ($H2O$, i.e. water) from the soil and carbon dioxide ($CO2$) from the air. The combined atoms of air and water as conveyed from the sun's energy form carbohydrates (COH). In our systems, these carbohydrates become the glucose that provides the primary energy to all of the cells of the body, including the brain. The glucose in the cell becomes the gradually liberated energy of the sun that sustains life itself.

The brain needs and uses approximately 40 percent of all consumed health-promoting raw carbohydrates. Among the most severe results of chronic lack of this necessary supply are digestive disturbances, fatigue, diminished concentration, impaired vision, excessive thirst, memory impairment and depression.

After more than 50 years of varied clinical research at The Institute, we have determined that at least 90 percent of every diet must consist of living vegan food, including sprouted grains, sprouted beans, vegetables (including their roots), and modest amounts of ripe, bio-organic fruit. This ideal diet of The Longevity Program assures excellent and consistent functioning of the brain and the rest of our systems.

All concentrated sugars — including white sugar, brown sugar, honey, maple syrup and others — are intense glycemic activators that cause rapid increases in blood-sugar levels, forcing the cells of the body that might already contain sufficient amounts of glucose to store this excess refined sugar. Inevitably, this leads to unhealthy weight increase, low blood sugar and diabetes.

Even the consumption of fruit must be monitored, because fruit has the same effect on the body as concentrated sugars; and all fruit must be completely avoided when you are in recovery from any disease. Dried fruits, for example, contain pure glucose, a substance that causes an immediate and severe increase of blood sugar.

Consume only those foods that release sugar slowly and safely into the bloodstream, allowing the body to use this fuel without disturbing health, functioning and concentration. Excess systematic sugar feeds and fuels viruses, bacteria, yeast, fungi, spirochetes, and the mutagenic agents that cause cancer.

All healthy uncooked carbohydrates other than those in fruits are formidable facilitators of the health of both body and brain. Without this solar-powered cuisine, your brain, body, life and functioning are depleted, damaged, debilitated and, sometimes, destroyed.

YOUR BEST SOURCES FOR GLUCOSE BALANCE:

The fueling of the brain requires the following appropriate complex carbohydrates: Sprouted grains, sprouted beans, root vegetables, and all green vegetables.

INTELLIGENCE-INDUCING NUTRIENTS: Vitamins, minerals and trace minerals facilitate both sustenance and improvement of brain, mind, thought and cognition. These critical nutrients turn glucose into energy, amino acids into neurotransmitters, simple fats into such complex forms as GLA, DHA and prostaglandins, and choline and serine into phosopholipids. This process builds and sustains the structure and substance of the brain.

A double-blind study, conducted in Europe by nutritionist Gwilym Roberts of England's Institute of Optimum Nutrition and psychologist Professor David Benton of Swansea University, revealed that the IQs of tested students who were given sufficient amounts of vitamins and minerals increased by 10 percent. As reported in the internationally respected British medical journal *Lancet*, the researchers concluded that consistent consumption of appropriate nutrients promotes and increases cognition, memory, concentration, and profundity and breadth of thought.

At a longevity conference in Paris, Dr. Domenica Rueff, author of several books on nutritional supplements, presented findings indicating that the stress placed upon the neurotransmitters of the brain (its "gray matter") can be reduced by consuming foods rich in selenium. The most essential complex of vitamins needed to promote, sustain and insure maximal brain functioning — thereby combating its cited deficiencies — is the B complex, the most important ones of which are these:

VITAMIN DEFICIENCIES' BEST RESOURCES:

1. For limited concentration and attention, Vitamin B 1, sprouted grains and green vegetables.

2. For depression, Vitamin B 3; for psychosis, sprouted grains and vegetables.

3. For memory deficiency, Vitamin B 5; for a deficient memory, wheatgrass; for stress, kamut grass and spelt grass.

4. For irritability, Vitamin B 6; for depression, sprouted quinoa; for memory loss and stress, sprouted amaranth and bananas.

5. For anxiety, folic acid; for depression, all the green sprouts; for psychosis, green leafy vegetables.

6. For confusion, Vitamin B 12; for psychosis, blue-green algae; for memory loss, green algae, sea vegetables and vegan B-12 supplements.

If any of the B vitamins are missing from your diet for any length of time, both thought and emotion are significantly impaired; obviously, therefore, you must have all of these B vitamins regularly to insure and promote maximum mental functioning. Since Vitamin C preceded all forms of life on Earth, it is clearly essential to all life, including the brain. Its primary function is to induce and maintain the balance of the neuro-transmitters in order to combat and reduce depression and schizophrenia. Those who suffer from these disorders need greater amounts of vitamin C. The best sources of which are sprouted garbanzo beans, red peppers, rose hips, acerola berry and amla.

Minerals and trace minerals build and maintain the structure of the brain, constituting and conducting its electrical current; without them, we would suffer mental, psychological and emotional difficulties.

BEST SOURCES FOR MINERAL
AND TRACE MINERAL DEFICIENCIES:

1. Anxiety and restlessness need the calcium found in juices of green vegetables and sprouts

2. Tension, fear, heart attacks, stroke, muscle pain and insomnia call for the magnesium found in sea vegetables, blue-green algae, green algae, kale, spinach, sprouted nuts and seeds.

3. Dizziness and convulsions can be helped by the manganese in sprouted nuts and seed and in tropical fruit.

4. Brain disfunction and immune system disorders respond to the selenium in sea vegetables, fresh water algae and bio dynamically grown vegetables.

5. Confusion, brain fog, depression, lack of motivation, impaired concentration and loss of appetite welcome sea vegetables, nuts and seeds.

YOUR BEST SOURCES OF
INTELLIGENCE-INDUCING NUTRIENTS:

You can literally broaden your mind, sharpen your wit, improve your cognition and maximize your thoughts by consuming the previously mentioned nutrients and the nourishing contents of the following brain banquet: All sprouted beans, all root vegetables, and avocados.

ANTIOXIDANTS: Many antioxidants are composed of the combination of vitamins and such elements as CoQ10 enzymes, alpha-lipoic acid, and others. As we have written, while oxidation erodes the brain, antioxidants combat that erosion by fighting free radicals (renegade electrons), which are the usual cause of the degeneration of brain and body.

Dr. Joel Pincemail of Belgium's University of Lieges maintains that a full supply of antioxidants is required for complete efficacy, because a limited supply cannot reach the sensitive essence of each cell, an essence that includes the mitochondries that produce most of our energy and are, consequently, most vulnerable to the assaults of the free radicals which are the primary cause of brain degeneration.

REMEMBER TO
PROTECT YOUR MEMORY

The results of comprehensive research involving the antioxidant content of 100 conventionally consumed "foods" were published in *The Journal of Agricultural and Food Chemistry*. The following "foods" were determined to have the best brain protective antioxidant content:

FRUITS, VEGETABLES, NUTS and SPICES: Cranberries, beans, pecans, cloves, blueberries, artichokes, walnuts, cinnamon, blackberries, sweet potatoes, hazelnuts, and oregano. These sources provide the best antioxidant brain protection; therefore, they must be regular parts of every healthy diet.

ENEMIES OF THE BRAIN

We have listed the allies of the brain. Let us now turn our attention to its enemies, all of which either are, cause, or become oxidants in the brain and body (please note that all these destructive elements wreak havoc on the highway and chaos at home, jeopardizing, impairing and devastating many thousands of lives every year).

ALCOHOL: Alcohol destroys brain cells, impairing cognition and memory. It sabotages the necessary 80 percent hydration of the brain by reducing its supply of essential water, obstructing the capacity and functioning of the cells of the brain (neurons). It also erodes and disintegrates the fatty acids that create and maintain the anatomical structure of the brain. During this destruction, alcohol also blocks the conversion of fats into DHA and prostaglandins, causing severely impaired mental functioning. Every alcoholic beverage disturbs, limits and destroys brain function and cognition.

TOBACCO: The catastrophically destructive effects of tobacco have been scientifically acknowledged for many years. Tobacco is unique among life's enemies because it is the most virulent airborne pollutant, poisoning not only its user but also those who are unfortunate enough to be nearby. The tobacco infestation caused by severely toxic second-hand smoke not only permanently harms but also kills hundreds of millions of people per year in North America alone.

Smoke — not only from cigarettes, but also from cigars, pipes, and marijuana (which we discuss in the next citation) — kills red blood cells, creating the free radicals that cause us to age prematurely. This vile despoiler of our air also reduces the level of oxygen in the bloodstream, crippling the immune system and ultimately causing every ailment from cancer to stroke to heart disease.

The noxious nicotine that is an ingredient in all tobacco products poisons the bloodstream, permanently impairing organ function, significantly reducing normal circulation, and dramatically inhibiting both sexual desire and sexual functioning.

A study conducted at North Carolina's prestigious Duke University revealed that the human body takes 17 smoke-free years before it can purge itself of the chronic effects of cigarette smoke. If you smoke, stop. Better yet? Never start.

If you have been — or still are — a chronic smoker, quit. In such circumstances, heed the advice of Dr. Thierry Souccar, a member of the Biology Society of Paris, who counsels people to have complete daily supplementation of whole-food vitamins C and E combined in order to avoid future vascular disease.

"RECREATIONAL" DRUGS: Among the many types of mind-altering and body-chemistry-altering drugs that are included under the misnomer of "recreational drugs" are marijuana, amphetamines, barbiturates, cocaine (including crack), opiates including heroin and opium, LSD and mescaline. Let's discuss each individually:

MARIJUANA: Despite the disclaimers by those who promote the medical use of marijuana, reputable studies have shown that smoking it produces three times greater susceptibility to contracting cancer than cigarettes. Smoking it also impairs response function, inhibits cognition, and destroys neurons.

AMPHETAMINES: These extremely dangerous man-made drugs alter the chemistry of both brain and body by artificially arousing and exhausting their ability to function. These fabricated addictive stimulants are often the cause of sleep deprivation, cardiovascular disorders, ventricle erosion, memory loss, sexual impairment and death.

BARBITURATES: These depressants numb brain function, causing lethargy, incoherence, speech impairment and decrease of mental functioning (destroying memory, distorting thought, and depriving the brain of its necessary oxygen). The narcotic effects of these drugs are often permanent, leading to respiratory problems, renal disorders, and the eradication of sexual desire and sexual potency. Clearly, "recreational drugs" are falsely named and truly dangerous.

COCAINE/CRACK: These singularly addictive killers alter brain chemistry and create a false sense of self that leads to erratic, dangerous, self-destructive behavior. They permanently alter the development of blood cells, distort the structure of bones and tissues, and attack cardiovascular functioning. Again, please note that although all of these "recreational" poisons are addictive, cocaine and crack are exceptionally so. So is heroin, about which we shall speak in the next listing.

OPIATES (heroin, opium): Opiates — among which the most extensively used and dangerous is heroin — deaden the senses and destroy both mental and physical functions. Chronic use of these extremely addictive toxins renders the user unfit both for normal social interaction and even minimal self-maintenance. The incessant ingestion of heroin causes the following permanent catastrophic effects: It impairs thought and creativity, destroys gastrointestinal function, sabotages both sexual desire and sexual performance, and alters vision and speech.

LSD AND MESCALINE: These hallucinogens are both natural and manmade; in either version, however, they not only distort perception but encourage paranoia, often rendering the user vulnerable and defenseless. Their use and abuse can cause permanent mental debilitation, psychiatric disorder, perpetual suspicion and a lack of self-confidence and coherent appreciation of reality.

TOXIC POLLUTANTS: The fumes generated by airborne pollutants such as tobacco smoke and chemical vapors (including everything from paint to perfume) also destroy brain cells, impairing mental function. These oxidants destroy the essential fats that create and sustain the structure of the brain by literally making them rancid and useless. This destructive process is often accompanied by fermentation that causes all types of headaches, including excruciating migraines. The vilest of oxidants is the smoke of tobacco and marijuana spewed from cigarettes, cigars and pipes; it harms everyone whom it assaults, whether first-hand or second-hand. Scientific estimates indicate that a single puff of any of these substances contains as many as one trillion — that's *1,000,000,000,000* — oxidants. This smoke also contains and emanates the heavy metal cadmium, which causes gradual depletion of the necessary zinc content of the brain. As we have noted, an insufficiency of zinc in the brain causes confusion, mind fog, loss of appetite, depression, limited concentration and lack of motivation.

HYDROGENATED FATS AND FRIED "FOODS": Most culpable among frequently consumed oxidants are the destructive so-called conventional "foods" ingested by billions of people. The molecular structure of these disease-causing enemies of brain, life and longevity is violated by the processing and heating of their oils. When they are processed and/or heated, they become indigestible and accumulate along arterial walls, within organs, and throughout the anatomy, causing diminished blood circulation, including its most essential component — oxygen.

As we have discussed, the most important fuel for the brain is glucose, which is a combination of $H2O$ and $CO2$. Another critical element of brain health is the oxygen independent of these combinations. Without a constant adequate supply of oxygen, the brain deteriorates to a point at which it eventually ceases to function, causing death.

STRESS: Stress causes distress. While the first two enemies of the brain are external chemical substances, stress is the internal saboteur that impairs brain function and restricts thought and mental potential. Under any kind of stress, levels of the hormone cortisol — one of the foremost antagonists of the brain's structure and functioning — increase. Research conducted at Stanford University by Dr. Robert Sapolsky has revealed that a mere two weeks of intense stress increases cortisol levels to the extent that they destroy dendrites, the connecting elements between brain cells. Although the dendrites are reinvigorated when cortisol levels decline, their functioning is impaired while stress is impinging upon them.

Of the various factors that cause premature aging, stress is the most virulent and prevalent. Our modern technological age oppresses us with the destructive, incessant, excessive stress that it imposes upon us at every chronological age. Researchers at La Sapienza University in Rome have discovered that the brains of the people who suffer from Alzheimer's disease have much higher levels of cortisol than the brains of those who are not thus impaired. In addition, the higher the cortisol level, the more pronounced the level of Alzheimer's disease.

At McGill University in Montreal, Dr. Linda Carlson and her colleagues have also confirmed that higher levels of cortisol cause increased memory loss. These scientists also discovered that sufficient amounts of the anti-stress hormone DHEA in the brain minimize cortisol's destructive effects on memory. Because of its importance to both mental functioning and longevity, let us discuss DHEA at greater length:

DHEA: THE ADRENAL HORMONE
THAT FIGHTS AND DEFEATS AGING

DHEA (Dehydroepiandrosterone) is essential not only to the control and limiting of stress; it is also pivotal in balancing the minerals that control the excessive production of sex hormones, which in turns facilitates the construction of lean body mass while combating the development of fat tissue. The levels of DHEA in the bloodstream determine the extent of one's aging process. Although all of the foods that we have mentioned promote and protect the body's supply of DHEA, damaged bodies might require whole-food supplementation of this precious hormone.

Most DHEA is produced in laboratories by means of genetic modification; obviously, these synthetic products must be avoided by everyone at every age. Herbal extracts of wild yam serve as a precursor of DHEA, increasing its bodily levels in a naturally healthy manner. Beneficial sources of DHEA are also available in homeopathic solutions.

GENERAL NUTRITION:
YOUR CONTINUED VITALITY

One of the most important assets for the maintenance of vitality and health is your choice of nourishing foods. There is no debate about which foods are the healthiest and most nutritious. Uncooked bio-organic fruits, vegetables, and germinated seeds, nuts, grains and beans constitute the essence of a wholesome diet. They are abundant with phytonutrients (natural chemistries) that prevent and eliminate disease. These living foods are packed with enzymes that fulfill the body's need for the electric charge that we continue to derive from the ultraviolet rays of the sun. Since our bodies are primarily electric, our trillions of red blood cells require constant reenergizing. The oxygen supplied by this vegetarian cuisine fills the cells with hemoglobin, intensifying clarity of thought and increased metabolic function. The hormones supplied by these powerful foods balance and improve the efficiency of the brain as well as the efficacy of the rest of the body.

NOURISHING YOUR LONGEVITY:
LONG LIFE — LESS FOOD

Studies published in *Proceedings of the National Academy of Science* show that eating small amounts of natural food and simply eating less food increase both health and longevity. It is important to note that limited consumption is particularly beneficial to seniors, who can increase their healthy life expectancy by 40 percent if they eat sensibly, exercise sufficiently, rest maximally and live vitally.

Research conducted and reported internationally indicates that our average life expectancy would be approximately 120 years if we ate appropriately by reducing our caloric intake.

One of the foremost authorities on life extension, Dr. Roy Walford of the Medical Center of the University of California at Los Angeles, established that health improves uniformly and comprehensively when we reduce food consumption.

All legitimate books about longevity indicate the importance of limited consumption for fulfilling longevity. Oxford University Press published *The Fountain of Youth: Culture, Scientific, and Ethical Perspectives on Biomedical Goals*, an anthology of contributions by experts in the areas listed in the book's title. In every discussion of the combination of diet and longevity, these renowned scientists emphasize the need for less eating to support more living.

Richard Weindruch, Ph.D., formerly of the National Institute of Health, conducted humane, non invasive and beneficial studies involving a great range of animals, including mammals. Each was provided with a more than adequate supplementation of all necessary nutrients, including vitamins, minerals, trace minerals, proteins, etc. Weindruch described this process as "undernutrition without malnutrition." The tested animals almost uniformly increased vitality, functioning and longevity (in some species, as much as 300 percent), along with reduction and/or healing of such serious diseases as cancer and auto-immune disorders.

ENERGY-CHARGED FOODS AND JUICES FOR YOUR LONGEVITY

Proper digestion is essential to proper nutrition. Most of the conventional "food" that we consume is difficult or impossible to digest. Our constant ingestion of this non-nutritive rubbish eventually debilitates and destroys us. Our depleted systems then must spend three full days using critical energy to eliminate the fragments of meat (all of which are non-digestible) from our bodies. The rancid residue of the consumption of this foul fodder is toxic cholesterol: animal fat, uric acid, other toxins and poisonous debris that clogs our physical network. This energy-destroying process dissipates our vitality, causing lethargy, depression and disease.

High-frequency bio-organic foods also provide exceptional nutrition in the easiest and most safely digested forms. The juices extracted from these foods provide us with abundant amounts of nutrients. Historically, chemists, nutritionists, biochemists and medical practitioners measured dietary proteins, vitamins, minerals and trace minerals to determine an individual's dietary deficiencies. Although these measurements are certainly important, they are not as essential to longevity as the amount of vibrational energy in each cell. At The Institute, we use microscopic analysis to determine the level of vibrancy of every cell of the body. Significant information is conveyed by this level of electrical energy.

You can increase your vibrational frequency through three basic methods:

1. Proper consumption of proper longevity-sustaining foods — one of the subjects of this chapter. Substances that provide the greatest nutritional benefits include those listed in the preceding paragraphs as well as enzymes, oxygen, hormones and phytochemicals, the elements that produce and sustain the function, energy and energy fields of our cells.
2. Daily consumption of pure nourishing liquids. Please see the chapter about hydration for information about this critical aspect of our nutrition.
3. Constructive interaction with nature (including other forms of life) as represented by the sun, fresh air and invigorating movement. Please read the other relevant sections of this book for additional discussion of these imperative contributions to longevity.

My own research continues to indicate that the following foods (categorized from Most to Medium to Modest in potency) are optimally effective in sustaining dynamic youthfulness.

MOST:

The foods in this group share the distinction of containing the highest levels of ultra violet vibrational activity directly from the sun: Tropical fruits such as mangos, cherimoya, sapote, caramboa, lichee, papaya. Green sprouts such as sunflowers, pea greens, fenugreek greens, clover, broccoli, turnips. Germinated grasses such as kamut, barley, spelt, wheat, rye, and fresh juices of all sprouts, including grasses and green coconut water.

MEDIUM:

This high-level maintenance banquet provides abundant levels of energy and helps sustain consistent physical and mental functioning: Non-tropical fruits such as grapes, apples, pears, peaches, plums, nectarines and cherries; fresh green vegetables like kale, mustard greens, broccoli, cabbage, lettuce, spinach, watercress and radicchio; familiar herbs such as parsley, coriander, watercress, basil, sage, rosemary and thyme; and fresh juices of green vegetables such as celery, cucumber, zucchini and other mentioned green vegetables.

MODEST:

At this level, you are sustained by a nutritional foundation that generates sufficient energy for basic activity: Hearty fruits such as persimmon, currants, cranberries, blueberries, cherries and gooseberries. Health-building nuts like almonds, filberts, pignolia, walnuts and pecans. Such seeds as pumpkin, sesame, flax, sunflower and hemp. Root vegetables like turnips, rutabaga, jicama, yucca and taro, and such root-vegetable greens as parsnip, turnip, mustard, collard and kohlrabi.

The exclusive and conservative consumption of foods from these three categories assures a long and healthy life. Those who need exceptional energy because of intensified physical, mental and emotional demands (including healing and recovery) should focus on foods in the Most classification. Those with a less demanding schedule can select offerings from the Medium range, and bodies at rest or reconstruction can be fueled and fulfilled by the items from the Moderate group.

The diet of those who are challenged by disease or under exceptional stress consists primarily of foods that have the greatest amount of ultraviolet frequency — with the exclusion of all fruits. I worked with a young man who had been diagnosed with fatal brain cancer. Allopathic practitioners had determined that conventional treatment had become irrelevant for him. When he arrived at Hippocrates, he was unable to sit for any length of time because of his deteriorating motor functions. Before he arrived he had been pharmaceutically sedated, leaving him disoriented and despondent. He proceeded to purge his system of the oppressive disease and destructive drugs that had depleted it. Slowly, with enormous determination, he reclaimed his life and re-created himself. He is now the father of two healthy children, and the entire family thrives with the healthy lifestyle that sustains his own longevity.

People who face such problems as diabetes, obesity and similar health concerns are benefited by foods in the Medium range — with the exception of fruits. Much of their distress has been caused by the ordinary "foods" they consumed, which have little or no vibrancy instead, they should — and can — easily graduate to the vibrationally fulfilling foods at the Medium level. A woman who weighed 400 pounds (180 kilograms) came to us oppressed by many health disorders caused by excess weight. The stress of that weight caused severe vital organ dysfunction, extreme chronic diabetes, dangerous immobility, constant pain, insufficient rest (including insomnia), and psychological anguish.

The Longevity Program provided her with almost immediate relief from all these life-threatening problems. Within three months, she had lost more than 100 pounds (50 kilograms). For the first time in decades, she was functioning efficiently, resting sufficiently, and living fully, paving the way for her healthy longevity.

Modest offerings are stepping-stones from miserable diets to the upper plateaus. Because they are heavier and therefore more filling, the items on the Moderate list appeal to those who are beginning The Longevity Program in order to improve body, mind and spirit. A young European came to us to help him prepare for the Olympic Games. As an athlete, he was accustomed to eating chemically laden, sugar-filled, non-nutritive junk. We provided him with nourishing, energy-sustaining real food and a positive environment! The discipline of his athletic regimen enabled him to improve not only his life but also his athletic performance — and to put both into perspective.

The fare in all three categories consists of uncooked cuisine of significant vibrational value. Once you have refined your health, functioning and awareness, your daily diet can include food from any of the three categories; however, your specific diet should be determined by your assessment of your physical and emotional situation, which you should consider every day.

All other so called "foods" fall below the Moderate designation; as such, they should be avoided.

For example, many people still believe that fish is healthy to eat. The stark reality is that all fish contain chemicals that are harmful to you. In the fishing port of Sete, France, many generations continue to buy the giant bass, mackerel, and eel that are at the poisonous bottom of the food chain. They should be made aware that these, and all other fish, are poisoned by the mercury that, when ingested, damages the human brain. These unfortunate sea creatures are also riddled by PCBs, dioxins and flame retardants, all of which are also toxic to the human system. All fish are now polluted, from ocean to ocean and sea to sea, including the once pristine Nordic waterways. Since the Industrial Revolution, we have managed to poison fish everywhere by throwing our industrial waste into our waters. Alarmed scientists and informed citizens have shown great concern about this catastrophic and systematic destruction of our waters and the creatures who dwell in them, but the situation may never be rectified because neither government nor industry is willing to address it. Instead, both continue to pursue and promote activities that ensure the continued degeneration of these essential life-serving elements of our planet.

San Francisco's Dr. Jane Hightower, lead researcher of a 21st-century study of mercury in medical patients, exposed this problem to international attention when she said, "As physicians, we are just starting to realize the effect of this chemical soup in which we all live. Each of us has to ask, 'Why are we poisoning ourselves?' " She noted that waters in many parts of the world are particularly dangerous because their contamination is trapped by ocean currents. "The Mediterranean is a toilet that no one has bothered to flush," Dr. Hightower said.

It is not only the Mediterranean that is at, and perhaps beyond, risk. More than 75 percent of the fish consumed by North Americans and Europeans is imported from countries that have either no governmental oversight or the most minimal of official involvement. That makes the problem truly — and troublingly — worldwide.

Kate Mahaffey, of the Environmental Protection Agency, has warned that even the most modest amount of toxin in fish can cause severe reactions in humans. Many people worldwide are contracting a form of mercury poisoning whose symptoms mimic cerebral palsy.

The journal *Nature* published a study that revealed the first comprehensive study of krill, the shrimp-like creatures once plentiful in our waters. Biologist Angus Atkinson, leader of the British Antarctic survey, says that krill are being replaced by salps, clear gelatinous invertebrates that provide almost no nutrition for their predators. Ecologists believe that this systematic displacement of krill from their natural habitats signals a major alteration of one of our most pristine and productive ecosystems. "We are just holding our breath to see what the consequences are," says William Fraser, another researcher of the Antarctic survey.

All our waters are polluted, which means that every form of life on the planet is threatened with extinction — and so is the planet's very essence. An example of this unconscionable development is the almost encyclopedic inclination of governments to promote industry at the expense of life in the world's waters, homes and human bodies.

One of the most outrageous examples of this lack of responsibility is the Environmental Protection Agency's intention to ally itself with the American Chemical Council to study the effect of pesticides on children. In a flagrant example of governmental irresponsibility and malfeasance, the EPA has bribed underprivileged families to exchange their children — including infants — for money. In exchange for $970, some clothing and a cheap video camera, these parents surrender their innocent, vulnerable children to two years of exposure to pesticides. This depraved lack of personal and governmental responsibility is especially heinous because it has been absolutely established that pesticides harm and kill people and other forms of life.

Research published in *The Journal of the National Cancer Institute* indicates that consuming biological/organically- grown vegetables and fruits protects and increases the health of our hearts. Other international studies have proven that these nutritious foods combat everything from mental illness to cancer.

Dr. Walter Willett of the Harvard School of Public Health has conducted an extensive 14-year study of the health of nurses — 72,000 women and 38,000 men. The study revealed that eating bio-organic fruits and vegetables increases immunity and helps the system resist the incursions of pesticides and fats that assault human health.

Implementation of The Longevity Diet assures you of the strongest immune system possible, which will facilitate your resistance to disease, increase your vitality, and prolong your life. We are meant to enjoy the pure, unpolluted vegetarian banquet of nature. If we adhere to this natural biological paradigm, we can add many healthy and vital years to our lives.

VIBRANT SUPERFOODS
THAT KEEP YOU VITAL

During the decades of my work involving nutrition, I have come to understand that the following four super-foods make up an excellent support system for a long and healthy life: Aloe vera, sea algae, fresh water algae, and flower and bee pollens are the most powerful vibrational allies your energized body has.

ALOE VERA

Research conducted both at The Institute and throughout the world proves that aloe vera is a distinguished contributor to vigorous life and longevity. Our research indicates that the hydrating qualities of aloe vera promote exceptional cell development by providing abundant amounts of healthy nutrients to every cell. The most essential ingredient for proper development of all organs — including the brain and the skin — is pure water. Aloe vera facilitates the absorption of 25 times more pure water into and throughout your cells. Since the body is primarily electric, the best conductor of its electricity is pure water. Consistent consumption of raw aloe vera (primarily in juice form) promotes and insures harmonious symbiotic interaction of electrons throughout your body. It is for this reason that, in the so-called burn wards found in hospitals throughout the world, aloe vera is immediately and regularly given to patients, both externally and internally.

Our research also indicates that the absorption of other nutrients is facilitated by their co-consumption with aloe vera. Aloe vera enhances proper digestion and elimination, and we have found it to be greatly beneficial in healing scar tissue and neutralizing its painful and unsightly effects. Oral administration and topical applications of this wonder plant also counteract the inflammation, irritation and scarring caused by chemotherapy and radiation. Extensive research conducted at the University of Pennsylvania indicates that this warm-weather plant can also be a viable temporary substitute in some cases of required blood transfusion, because it can keep organs alive for several hours.

Aloe vera is also aesthetically viable because it is the best natural moisturizer for your skin at any age, whether taken internally or applied externally. If you consume $1/22^{nd}$ liter (one ounce) of raw aloe vera daily, you will achieve and maintain the long healthy life that you deserve.

SEA ALGAE

These saltwater power-plants are the foods that invigorate and sustain Earth's largest creature — the blue whale. The earth's richest soil is at the bottom of our oceans. The forests of seaweed that grow from this nutritious source are rich with minerals and trace minerals. These elements are the conductors of the electric frequency within each cell and from cell to cell. Appropriately, the minerals of the intestinal tract are, in fact, called electrolytes.

Our various coastlines — from France's Brittany to Ireland's Donegal, from Canada's province of Nova Scotia to the expansive coastline of China — provide many nutritious seaweeds for harvesting and consumption.

Some of the most readily available seaweeds are arame, dulse, hijiki, nori and wakame, but there are many others. Proteins (amino acids) are also plentiful in these foods. The uncooked form of each possesses a unique combination of vitamins, hormones, oxygen, phytochemicals and enzymes. The brain, cardiovascular system, nervous system, respiratory system, endocrine system, and circulatory system all benefit from the consumption of these vital gifts of nature.

Sea algae enhance vision and hearing, two senses that most commonly degenerate with age. The calming effect of these powerful plants is both internal and external, so bathing in their extracts and enjoying seaweed baths and seaweed wraps nourish and exhilarate body, mind, emotions and spirit.

FRESH WATER ALGAE
(BLUE-GREEN AND GREEN)

These single-cell powerhouses of vitality constitute the first life on earth, and their development and functions are unique. They are the most protein-rich foods, consisting of more than 50 percent complete and digestible amino acids as well as essential vitamins and many minerals and trace minerals.

Throughout the decades, we have supplemented The Longevity Program with blue-green and/or green algae, because they have proven to strengthen the constitutions of both the healthy and the healing. They support the DNA that is the building block of each body. Fresh water algae are essential to potent longevity.

International research proves that blue-green algae activate and create stem cells, which are the generators of all other cells; stem cells help rebuild the tissues of the liver, the nervous system, the brain, and every other part of the body.

Green algae — also called chlorella — benefit those who suffer from blood-sugar disorders, and these super-nutrients assist the removal of heavy metals and radioactive materials from the body. Green algae were the primary supplements I used successfully in my work with victims of Chernobyl.

At The Institute, we continue to help people rid themselves of heavy metal toxins with the use of chlorella. The consumption of these powerful plants helps to regulate both low blood sugar (hypoglycemia) and high blood sugar (diabetes). Taking five tiny pills of chlorella every two to four waking hours for as long as necessary helps to regulates blood sugar effectively.

Green and blue-green algae build both hemoglobin and the rest of the red blood cell, providing the brain with the natural fatty acids it requires for its constant reconstruction, renewal and regeneration. They also help vitalize your organs and muscles, giving them greater strength, elasticity and durability. These anti-aging miracles should be part of your daily self-rejuvenating diet.

FLOWER AND BEE POLLENS

Flower pollens are pellets of energy gathered from flowers, pellets so powerful they are able to sustain essential life. The Royal Science of the Naturalists of Mons, in Belgium, and Borinage, in France, published *The Secret Life of Bees*, which lists many of the essential nutrients in both flower and bee pollens; among these are Vitamins A, B-1, B-2, B-6 and E, Vitamin C, inositol, pantothenic acid, nicotinic acid, essential amino acids, arginine, histenine, leucine, lysine, methionine, isoleucine, phenylenylalanine, phreonine, tryptophan, and valine. This book notes that pollens contain these minerals as well as the trace minerals potassium, magnesium, calcium, copper, iron, silicone, phosphorous, sulphur, chlorine, and manganese. Other elements in pollens are biotin, folic acid, lactoflavine, and the soil-based probiotic known as B-12.

The combination of these powerful nutrients combats the damaging effects of free radicals that cause many of the symptoms and problems of deteriorating aging. Pollens also reduce and eliminate allergies, enhance the immune system and strengthen every cell, tissue and membrane of the body.

The daily consumption of one tablespoon or soupspoon of bee or flower pollen helps maintain vital, energetic life and longevity.

NUTRITION THAT KEEPS YOU SUPPLE

Living whole-food supplements promote the development of a strengthened anatomy. Obviously, supplements cannot provide all of your necessary nutrition. Therefore, you must combine them with the energizing diet and lifestyle provided by The Longevity Program, because every part of your body must be constantly sustained by those 10 trillion healthy cells.

The largest organ — the skin — is the protective membrane surrounding this system; consequently, the condition of your skin is a reliable and critical indicator of overall health. Smooth, clean and unblemished skin is external indication of apparently good health. Physiognomy (analysis of the face, eyes and nails) is used to assess the degree of health of internal organs.

A person who achieves the highest level of health by means of proper living, diet, exercise and interaction is often described as "glowing." This glow is actually caused by the positive electrical charge flowing throughout the body and emanating from the person. Properly nourished and well-hydrated organs that function at maximum frequency embody and emit a healthy electrical charge. Allopathic practitioners can measure your physical health electromagnetically by using such diagnostic tools as Magnetic Resonant Imagery (MRI), high-speed CAT Scans and PET scans. Unfortunately, they then often treat you with commercial pharmaceuticals.

The body requires constant reinvigoration from living food that sustains and renews the life force. Advanced technology has already started to measure our health and longevity by the amount of electrical frequency that we generate, maintain and utilize. The Longevity Program provides the simplest, easiest and most effective way to achieve a healthy long life. The most reliable measure of your degree of health is determined by the following six-level standard, going from the depths of darkness to the beauty of brilliance, which we at The Institute created.

DARKNESS

Menu	The Body	The Mind
Meat; dairy; baked goods; cooked "food"; synthetic "food";	Inactivity; injuries; abuse; illness;	Negativity; fear; hostility; restriction

ECLIPSE

Menu	The Body	The Mind
Lacto-ovo vegetarian "food"; non-bio-organic fare;	Limited activity; recovery and renewal; healing	Frustration; timidity; anger

SHADOW

Menu	The Body	The Mind
Lacto-vegetarian and bio-organic fare	Flexibility and increased strength	Skepticism; sarcasm

CLOUDS

Menu	The Body	The Mind
Mostly bio-organic living food; fresh juices	Full initiation of aerobic and resistance exercise	Calm; clever; trusting; functional

LIGHT

Menu	The Body	The Mind
Predominantly bio-organic living food; wheatgrass-juice; sprout-juice	Flexibility; resilience; athleticism; endurance	Confidence; creativity; courage; calm

BRILLIANCE

Menu	The Body	The Mind
Pure bio-organic living-food diet, including power-juices and algae daily; weekly fasting	Full aerobic and resistance exercise; maximum strength and flexibility; complete health optimal rest	Activity; acuity; insight; knowledge; understanding; comprehension

At your own pace, in your own time, you should aspire to achieve the greatest possibility. Many of us undertake the journey of life in darkness, seeing nothing, and acting accordingly. This haphazard voyage hurts not only the traveler but also those against whom he collides in the darkness. At this vulnerable level it is easy to be manipulated because, in the dark, one has no direction – but while making a lifetime's journey without vision is difficult, a life without conscious awareness is infinitely worse. Everyone needs to advance toward the light, and the vehicle for doing so is self-respect, because self-respect is the foundation of maturity and the cornerstone of longevity.

For more than half a century, The Hippocrates Health Institute has contributed to the improvement of the human condition. We have helped people find their way out of darkness, out of eclipse, out of shadow, and beyond clouds into the brilliant light of the life luminously lived.

The process is gradual for most people. And there is nothing wrong with periodic sojourns backwards as long as the direct path is always forward. We are fortunate to have formidable assistance for our journey. For example, we have anti-aging herbs, sprouts and other nutrients to help keep us young. Here is a list of some of their greatest benefits:

ALPHA-LIPOIC ACID (ALA)
The Italian whole food ALA is a powerful antioxidant that helps protect the body from free-radical damage. It also reinvigorates Vitamins C and E, affording you increased protection from free radicals. It lowers cholesterol, protects nerve tissue, detoxifies the liver by eliminating heavy metals from it, and strengthens the cells of the immune system.

BILBERRY
This herb helps to preserve vision and prevent degenerative eye disease. It also balances circulatory functioning and strengthens the tissues of the cardiovascular system.

CABBAGE SPROUTS
It is best to germinate cabbage seeds, thereby maximizing the phytochemical effect of the sulphur compounds in this member of the cruciferous vegetable family. The consumption of germinated cabbage seeds helps combat digestive and eliminatory disorders. It also fights ulcers and minimizes or even eliminates arthritic and osteoporotic conditions. It is also a significant contributor in the prevention and elimination of various cancers.

DAIKON RADISH
This Asian radish is known for its blood-purifying properties and its mineral-rich nutritive powers, both of which help the body to maintain vitality and healthy functioning.

ELDERBERRY
The seeds of this fruit enhance the capacity of the neurons (brain cells), enabling the brain to function efficiently and clearly. They also energize the eye's iris and help to improve and sustain your vision.

FENNEL-SEED SPROUTS
Germinating this seed increases its potency. Fennel seed assists digestion and combats esophageal disorders. It also stimulates the development of sperm and healthy ovarian secretions. This hormone-strengthening sprout helps sustain sexual and all other vitality.

GABA
(GAMMA AMINOBUTYRIC ACID)
This stimulating natural amino acid helps your body produce human-growth hormones that prevent degenerative aging. Declining levels of these hormones can cause many of the symptoms associated with unhealthy aging, including weight gain, muscle loss, reduced energy, insufficient sleep, aging of skin, loss of bone density, and libidinal decline.

HORSETAIL
(EQUISETEUM ARVENSE)
This herb contains significant amounts of natural silicone, one of the first minerals usually lost to aging. Your bones, skin, cartilage, connective tissues, hair, and arteries are strengthened by regular consumption of horsetail, which prevents the unnecessary loss of natural silicone.

INDIAN HEMP
(CANNABIS SEEDS)
This variety of hemp is known for the nutritious value of its seeds which, when sprouted, become one of the best sources of omega oils (fatty acids). Balanced levels of Omega-3 and Omega-6 enhance the immune system, the cardiovascular system and brain functioning.

JERUSALEM ARTICHOKE
This root vegetable member of the sunflower family contains a unique form of complex carbohydrates that has the capacity to regulate blood sugar. Stable levels of blood sugar enhance longevity by reducing both the physical and the functional stress on all of the vital organs, including the brain, as well as the nervous system.

KOHLRABI

This root is a member of the cabbage family. Its sulphur content benefits every system of the body. It counteracts bone disorders of the legs and feet, and its anti-mutagenic properties combat cancer.

LAMINERIA

This Asian kelp assists the functioning of the glands (especially the thyroid), the function of which is to create, regulate and balance hormones. The most significant deterrent to premature aging is the retention of hormonal vitality.

MILK THISTLE
(SILYBUM MARIANUM)

Silymarin, an active ingredient in milk thistle, stimulates the regeneration of liver cells. It protects and repairs the liver, an organ that serves the body in more than 500 ways. Proper liver function is essential to a long, healthy life.

NUTMEG

The powdered form of this tasty herb can be added to foods and drinks. In all its forms, it benefits nerve development, enhances circulatory functioning, and increases male sexual potency.

ONION SPROUTS

Sprouted onion seeds help to prevent abnormal growths in and on the body, including cysts, fibroid tumors and mutagenic cancers. They also enhance bone density and reduce the possibility and the occurrence of acne. *The British Journal of Medicine* has reported that onions are 25 percent more effective than Fosamax in strengthening bones and teeth.

PEA GREENS

These sprouted baby pea plants are filled with protein (amino acids) that help build muscle, cells and strength. They also facilitate the functioning of the spleen, gallbladder and urinary tract. These sprouts are essential to The Longevity Program.

QUINOA

This grain has historically been cultivated by the natives of South America. Its mineral content and protein content give it great prominence as an architect and custodian of every part of the body. Its uncooked and sprouted form alkalizes the system, protecting it from disease.

RUTABAGA GREENS

Planted in potted soil and watered daily, this root vegetable produces green leaves throughout the year; these plants can be harvested and juiced and/or added to salad. Rutabaga greens benefit the sinuses, the respiratory system and the stomach, parts of the body that tend to degeneration and untimely aging.

STRING BEANS

Raw or juiced, string beans are rich in both minerals and trace minerals. They help build and protect nerves, white blood cells, hair and valves.

TURMERIC (CURCUMA LONGA)

Curcumin, the active ingredient in turmeric, is effective in suppressing pain in the same way as pharmaceuticals such as COX 1 and COX 2 inhibitors. Turmeric is a powerful ally against many types of pain and inflammation associated with aging. Combating memory loss is it's greatest asset

UVA URSA (BEARBERRY)

This fascinating sprout is known as the "upland cranberry." A low evergreen shrub, its seed is dried and then sprouted for three days. A diuretic, astringent, and mucilage antiseptic disinfectant, its root and leaves provide relief for bladder congestion, kidney congestion and backache, as well as the symptoms and problems associated with the prostate and with gonorrhea and syphilis. It also eliminates excess mucus, helps the body resist microbial infection, and promotes a sense of hopefulness and security.

VALERIAN ROOT

In its herbal form, Valerian is a mild sedative that helps to reduce pain and assist sleep. Insomnia might be the most prevalent oppressor of those in their mature years. Sleep deprivation can actually be deadly, but we need to fight it only by natural means, of which Valerian is one of the best.

WATERMELON SEED SPROUTS

These succulent protein-rich plants reach full growth in seven days. They provide minerals that ensure the elasticity of body tissue, as well as providing proteins that build cells, and nutrients that enhance the function of the kidneys, bladder and lungs.

XANTHIUM (XANTHIUM STRUMARIUM; COCKLEBUR)

This herb grows in China, Japan, Korea, Taiwan, and various parts of Europe. Its roots, stems, hairy leaves, and fruits are used in traditional Asian medicine to combat the common cold, headaches, German measles, and other diseases and illnesses. Using the dried seed, and sprout for three days. Its seed helps to combat hepatitis, colds, flu, SARS, and other microbial infections. It also confers confidence.

YELLOW SQUASH

This warm-weather squash possesses nutrients that benefit vision, hearing and other sensory functions. In addition, it corrects abnormal menstruation. Its capacity to strengthen both male and female hormones makes it a powerful ally of potent longevity.

ZINGIBER OFFICINALE
(JAMAICAN GINGER ROOT)

Ginger root planted in organically fertilized potted soil and watered daily sprouts a stalk and yields a green sprouted shoot that can be cut for juicing or for immediate consumption; it must be consumed before it is 5 centimeters (3 inches) high. Zingiber balances hormones and regulates the body's internal thermometer and its natural thermostat, keeping us cool as necessary; it contains potent anti-cancer and anti-viral chemistries as well as combats microbes and mutagens. Jamaican ginger root helps alleviate motion sickness. This root is conventionally known as Jamaican ginger.

PRACTICAL LONGEVITY:
EASY WAYS TO STAY YOUNG

As humanity has aged, we have developed many easy dietary means to facilitate functioning and promote longevity. Following are some of the best methods — listed by the parts and functions of the body that they benefit — to sustain yourself in your natural effort to combat unnatural aging:

BRAIN: Hemp seeds: These nutritious seeds provide all the fatty acids that your body needs and your brain requires for reconstruction and sustenance. The complete proteins in them help enhance focused thought and vigorous creativity. They also stabilize intestinal balance, promoting the creation of enough serotonin to nourish the brain.

SKIN, SCALP, HAIR, BONES: Lemon grass and horsetail. These healing herbs can be converted into living sun tea by soaking them in two ounces (60 milliliters) or one quart (one liter) of pure water. Both contain concentrations of silica that promote hair growth and strengthen both the soft and hard tissues of the body, from bones to skin including the scalp.

EYES, INTESTINES: The cabbage family. There is a fascinating but absolute connection between your eyes and your intestines: They are both positively affected by the potent sulphur compounds in the cabbage family. These nourishing plants contain considerable amounts of beta carotene, which sustain and strengthen every part of the eyes. Members of the cabbage family help your intestines to secrete and regulate the gastric fluids necessary for proper organ function.

EARS, CARDIOVASCULAR SYSTEM: Cayenne pepper (Capsicum). This potent pepper prevents circulation impairment, one of the primary causes of tinnitus and excess accumulation of ear wax. Cayenne pepper stimulates the bloodstream, purifying the heart and its thousands of miles of tributaries. Prostate cancer cells cannot survive with capsicum.

MOUTH, ESOPHAGUS, NECK, HEART: Garlic contains antibiotic and antimicrobial potency that kills the microbes and spirochetes that inhabit the mouth and the pathways, including the neck, to which it is a conduit. These vermin are the causes of many diseases, and garlic is one of the best herbal preventives against them.

LUNGS AND THE REST OF THE RESPIRATORY SYSTEM: Eucalyptus (bio-organic), a beneficial oil that can be taken orally to strengthen and purify both the lung's tissues and functioning, thus combating asthma, emphysema, and the cancers that attack this system.

BREASTS AND OTHER PECTORAL COMPONENTS: Mung bean sprouts are filled with zinc and other minerals that cleanse and purify the lymph glands, purging them of toxins that assault the chest and cause lymphatic infections and cancer.

HEART; VENTRICLE SYSTEM: Raw artichokes can be juiced or eaten raw. This vegetable's nutrients help build veins and capillaries, regulate and empower heart function, and reduce the accumulation of catarrh. Once cooked, the residue can be combined with raw aloe vera gel to serve as a poultice for bruises, varicose veins and burst capillaries.

KIDNEYS; BLADDER: Melons and cucumbers contain concentrations of mineral and water that create the alkalinity needed for renal organs to function properly, thereby purging the body of impurities. They also help facilitate blood flow throughout the renal system.

LIVER; GALLBLADDER; MUCUS MEMBRANES: Beet and collard greens, both raw and juiced, increase the number of red blood cells, intensify the activities of H-cells and fighter cells (immune system agents), and cleanse the liver and gallbladder.

STOMACH; SMALL INTESTINE: Flaxseeds. Among the many foods benefiting the digestive system, flaxseeds help it to purge itself of impurities while simultaneously strengthening its form and functioning with powerful proteins.

LARGE INTESTINE; BOWELS; ANUS; RECTUM: Turnip-root juice stabilizes intestinal balance and builds the tissues of the large intestine, the bowels, and the rectal area. It can be used either by drinking or bowel implantation.

LOWER BACK; HIPS; SKELETON: Sea vegetables; their calcium and magnesium strengthen and renew bone structure and stabilize the spine, hips, back, and all the body's bones.

GENITALIA OF BOTH SEXES: Lettuce (especially iceberg lettuce). As the source of life, our genitalia must be given life-sustaining nutrition. The opiate effect of lettuce enhances libido, promotes blood circulation throughout the genital area, and fights and neutralizes prostate problems and vaginal infections.

LEGS (including thighs, knees, calves, ankles and feet): Celery or celery root, whose organic sodium and minerals benefit circulation in the lower extremities, reducing the occurrence or minimizing the impact of phlebitis, neuropathy and related conditions.

CHAPTER FIVE

HYDRATION: PARTAKE OF THE FOUNTAIN OF YOUTH

Almost 85 percent of the human brain consists of water, and our bodies are 75 percent water. Clearly, plenty of pure water is necessary for a healthy life. However, dehydration devastates the mental and physical functioning of millions of people each year. Dehydration causes an imbalance of electrolytes (minerals), mimicking the symptoms of senility, demonstrating all too clearly the importance of proper hydration.

Not only are most of us dehydrated, but even those who drink sufficient liquid are endangered by the international epidemic of poisonous water. Our oceans, lakes, rivers, streams and ponds are polluted by heavy metals, acid rain, garbage dumps, industrial waste and agricultural debris. As a result, according to environmental researcher and explorer, the late Jacques Cousteau, hundreds of thousands of deaths every year are attributed to arsenic poisoning, which causes a slow and painful degeneration, maiming the victim limb by limb and organ by organ. Toxicity caused by heavy metals such as mercury is directly linked to many deadly diseases, including cancer, Parkinson's disease, Amyotrophic Lateral Sclerosis (Lou Gehrig Disease), and some forms of mental illness.

Brain-altering toxins cause memory loss, decreased motor function, even cardiovascular distress. We must enrich our bodies — especially our brains — with pure water, rather than deplete and destroy them with toxic liquids.

Alcohol and coffee dehydrate the body and weaken the immune system. The alleged benefits of wine to increase life span are misguided and false. The fact is that alcohol destroys cells — especially in the brain and other vital organs. Whatever benefit is ascribed to wine is instead derived from the grapes used to make it. According to researchers at Johns Hopkins University, it is actually the astringency of grape skins that reduces inflammation in the veins, thereby reducing the potential for heart attacks and strokes.

The carbonation of so called "soft drinks" reduces the oxygen supply throughout the body, interfering with the natural functioning of all anatomical and metabolic systems. Studies in Britain and elsewhere indicate a direct correlation between the consumption of soda and excess weight. The health-promoting function of pure water is twofold: It hydrates the cells and tissues of the body as well as cooling and moisturizing the skin.

Bathing is also an essential aspect of hygienic self-hydration. Not only does warm water feel good, it relaxes the nervous system, regulates and balances organ functions, soothes the spirit and, of course, cleanses and purifies the body by removing most of the one kilogram (two pounds) of waste eliminated daily through the skin. High-pressure baths such as whirlpools and Jacuzzis provide additional stimulation to the lymphatic system and vital organs, increasing circulation, detoxification, immunity and relaxation.

Water vapor, steam baths, Russian and Turkish baths help detoxify the lungs, kidneys and bladder. Smokers, former smokers and those who have been exposed to smoke and other kinds of pollution derive great benefit from these water-based therapies.

Dry saunas and Far-infrared saunas remove toxins from the liver, the gallbladder, and the vascular system. Dry saunas work from the outside in, Far-infrared saunas the inside out, but since both cause water to evaporate from your body it is essential for you to drink sufficient amounts of pure water during and after every sauna. Researchers at Stockholm's Karolinska Hospital have reported that effective saunas provide benefits similar to those derived from aerobic exercise.

There are pure fluids other than water that can nourish and invigorate your body. Raw green-vegetable juice and sprout juice are the most effective and nutritious sources of natural hydration. Small amounts of ripe bio-organic fruit and vegetable juices also provide you with essential nutrients. Mineral-rich juices are the most productive sources of basic hydrating elements for your body's cells. The nutrients in these juices help conduct the positive electricity of vital energy that travels throughout your system.

The internal and external use of pure water is essential to healthy longevity. Ironically, as we age, many of us reduce our fluid consumption. Ironically, too, as Earth ages, our water becomes increasingly impure. The water that was part of Earth at its beginning is the water that is part of it now and forever. We have contaminated our waters with toxic chemicals since the Industrial Revolution, and we continue to do so at an alarming rate. Infectious disease is epidemic throughout the world because microbes, parasites and amoebae breed in our polluted waters. In many parts of the world, the major cause of death is consumption of liquids from contaminated water sources.

More specifically, in Europe and North America many deaths are caused by the chemical contamination of air and water. In developing nations, most deaths result from the biologically destructive microbes and parasites that inhabit that air and water. As time passes, these contaminating elements will combine to wreak ever more catastrophic death and disturbance of nature. They are even more deadly in combination than they are individually.

Japanese technologists created a method by which both biological and chemical sources can be filtered out of our water while, at the same time, creating a vortex that organizes the water's molecules. My research at The Institute, involving thousands of people, has demonstrated that the consumption of this water increases the electromagnetic charge in and around body cells, preventing free-radical damage. (Free radicals are the primary cause of premature aging and disease.) In addition to preventing damage by free radicals, this water generates greater electromagnetic frequency in the cells, creating a reserve of physical and mental energy.

We conducted a focus study involving bottled water harvested from a mountain that houses a potentially active volcano. This water includes a natural high-energy component that derives from the heat and pressure of molten lava. For three weeks, 23 of our residents — each of whom had a catastrophic disease indicating a fatal prognosis — drank only this water (Nariwa) in conjunction with the living-food program at Hippocrates.

When we compared their progress to those of 23 other residents who were similarly afflicted, our findings indicated that the immune function of those who consumed Nariwa had been increased by 18.5 percent.

Pure water is quickly becoming the most endangered of our many endangered precious resources. Residents of privileged countries have been buying bottled water for decades; the less fortunate have been drinking and bathing in polluted waters for years. What was once the abundant, pure gift of nature could become the source of armed conflict, including global war.

In order to avoid this catastrophe, we must stop polluting our resources. Morality and ethics aside, survival dictates that we do so.

It is clear that the invisible elements in our water can either help or hurt us. Each of us is responsible for ensuring that we consume adequate amounts of clean, healthy water daily. Nothing is more important to good health than pure water.

A DAY WITH YOUR LONGEVITY-PROGRAM DIET

The following is one of many possibilities of a day's diet to support your longevity:

BREAKFAST:
Begin your invigorating day with fresh juice containing either bio-organic fruit and pure water or a drink made of green vegetables and/or watermelon rinds and/or sprouts. After breakfast, take your primary supplements, tailored to your individual needs. At the beginning of your adaptation to The Longevity Program, you may require additional nutrition: when you do, you can eat either cereal or bread made from sprouted grains, although many people prefer raw salads instead.

MID-MORNING JUICE OR TEA BREAK:
If possible, have a fresh drink of green vegetables and sprouts. If you cannot do so, have uncooked sun tea warmed at temperatures below 115 degrees Fahrenheit or 42 degrees Celsius.

LUNCH:

Begin with a large glass of pure water or fresh non-sugary vegetable juice. Wait 15 to 30 minutes, then eat a large green salad and any of the following: Loaves and patties made of nuts and seeds; mixed salads made of sprouted beans and/or grains; cooked whole grain pasta; steamed vegetables; other choices from the great range of internationally available vegetarian/vegan cuisine.

MID-AFTERNOON JUICE BREAK OR TEA BREAK:

If possible, have a fresh green drink consisting of green vegetables and sprouts. If you cannot do so, have uncooked sun tea that is warmed at temperatures below 115 degrees Fahrenheit or 42 degrees Celsius.

DINNER:

Dinner should involve raw vegetarian foods that are lighter than those of your lunch. When you have finished your dinner, you have finished your day's eating. However, you can drink healthy fluids until two hours before you retire. It is necessary to desist from drinking at least two hours before sleeping so that your system does not need to process liquids during the night, thereby disturbing your sleep. You can alter this suggested dietary regimen as necessary, depending upon your emotional and physical circumstances.

Above all, you must eat well to live long, because positive longevity depends upon a healthy diet. Fail to eat well and you cannot live well. The fuel for a productive long life is given us by nature; let us welcome that gift and use it to our advantage. Nothing you do will reach full fruition if your diet is deficient, so to fulfill your goals and enjoy long life you must also fulfill your nutritional needs.

CHAPTER SIX

EXERCISE: MOVE TO FLOURISH

Your mind needs productive and positive activity; your body needs energizing and exhilarating exercise. Age is no barrier to either, for each supports the other at every age. The following three basic kinds of exercise are available to everyone of every age:

1. Stretching: Stretching before and after exercise is always important; however, it becomes more essential as the years proceed. Stretching-enhanced flexibility benefits all activities, including exercise, regulation and stimulation of all bodily systems, creation of the endorphins that minimize depression and anxiety, and optimal rest. In order to be mobile, you need a limber body. The body is the vehicle of our journey through life, so we need to treat it well. Constant counterproductive movements and activities prevent the body from unrestricted functioning, inhibiting its freedom of movement and activity. If you stretch before and after every exercise, you will attain maximal flexibility and fluidity with minimal injury and degeneration.

2. Aerobics: Aerobic exercise has two functions: to activate and strengthen all bodily systems, and to detoxify the body by helping it eliminate waste. Research at The Institute has proven that proper and adequate aerobic exercise helps remove waste and combats disorders eight times faster than if no exercise is done. Aerobic exercise is a critical component of fulfilled and fulfilling longevity.

Based on a study of 4,835 participants, researchers at Long Island Jewish Medical Center determined that certain times are better for exercise than others. The worst times are early morning and midday, because lung function is least expansive at those times. The best are late morning and early evening, when lung functioning is at its maximum and our biological cycles are at maximum pitch. These conclusions are based on the circadian rhythms that naturally govern human activity.

3. Resistance exercise: The strength and durability of both your skeleton and your muscles are enhanced by resistance exercise; in fact, without resistance exercise for a considerable length of time the body atrophies and loses most of its muscle tone. Resistance exercise offers you the opportunity to lift weight against gravity, salvaging you from gravity collapsing your weight — so lift weights instead of letting them hang from you. Resistance exercise helps to prevent osteoporosis, back pain, skeletal deformities and degeneration, arthritis, rheumatism, and loss of memory.

At every age, the best bodies need and use all three of these forms of exercise. International research — including that done by Terrie Fox Wetle of the Gerontological Society of America — indicates that more than one-third of those over 65 do no regular health-promoting physical activity, and two-thirds of those people do not eat the minimally required five servings of fruits and vegetables per day. Just as frightening? They also consume slightly more requisite nutrients than the rest of the population.

Studies have also shown that obesity is rampant not only around the world but also among seniors, more than 30 percent of whom suffer from excessive weight and weight gain. All forms of proper exercise promote health and longevity; even regular walks can cut memory loss by as much as 50 percent. Dr. Everett Koop, former Surgeon General of the United States and an authority on Alzheimer's disease, suggests that weightlifting stimulates various parts of the brain, thereby supporting its vitality and functioning.

Consistently performed healthy exercise provides us with joy, vigor, enthusiasm and energy. Let us review the three listed essential forms of exercise: stretching, aerobic and resistance.

Both ancient and modern forms of exercise benefit the body. For example, Pilates and some forms of yoga have threefold benefits: Flexibility, increased muscle mass, and improved focus and relaxation.

Swimming, speed walking, in-line skating, dancing, cross-country skiing, bicycling, and rowing are of great benefit to the cardiovascular system, including the heart, and in the elimination of bodily toxins. Our modern world gives us access to such indoor aerobic wonders as elliptical equipment, Stairmasters, treadmills, stationary bicycles, mechanical rowing machines and many others. A minimum of 35 minutes of aerobic exercise five days a week is necessary for every capable person of any age to sustain health, endurance, strength and vigor.

Hatha yoga, non-competitive gymnastics, callinetics, weight- bearing equipment, free weights, water-based weight resistance and other exhilarating activities all utilize forms of resistance exercise. Exercise benefits not only your body but also your self-confidence; it helps you to not only feel your best but to be your best and look your best. Your attractive mature self generates confidence and positive energy. A conventional stigma attached to aging is that anatomy weakens within you, around you and beyond you. Not only is this not true, but the strength and visual appeal of every body can be sustained throughout its maturity.

Dr. Jean Meyer, former president of Tufts University, who compared the physical condition of healthy centenarians to that of young athletes, found that those aged 100 or more can build muscle in a manner similar to the development of teenage Olympians.

A prime example of this, and a testament to positive attitude, proper living, and healthy exercise for almost a century, is Jack LaLanne, born September 26, 1914. Other mature masters of life include Jeanne Calment, who lived productively for 122 years, remaining active, curious, creative, positive and healthy throughout. Christian Mortensen lived 110 years of joy, vigor and vitality. Among the many others of similarly rewarding longevity are Habib Miyan (approximately 125 years), Shige Chiyo (121 years), and Irving Berlin (101 years). Verona Johnston (114 years) interrupted her activities just long enough to summarize the importance of exercise: "When you keep moving, they can't put you into a box." As you see, these three types of primary exercise are necessary at every age, so you must do each of them to whatever degree possible according to your health, schedule and preferences.

CHAPTER SEVEN

SLEEP AND OTHER FORMS OF REST: RECONSTITUTE YOUR ESSENCE

Lost sleep is lost life: If you cannot sleep when you should, you will doze when you should be active and sleepwalk through your days. Healthy adults require about 8 hours of uninterrupted sleep each night. Based on metabolism, genetics and individual situations, the acceptable range varies from a minimum of seven hours to a maximum of nine. Researchers at the University of Buffalo and elsewhere have reported that lost sleep has catastrophic cumulative effects. The loss of just one hour of sleep each night costs the average adult an accumulated 365 hours a year. This deprivation also impairs waking hours, because attention, concentration, thought, work, and play are damaged.

Sadly, many adults lose far more than a single hour of sleep each night. Some suffer with deprivations of as much as three or four hours a night, while others can hardly sleep at all, and a severe loss of sleep shortens life.

The American Cancer Society conducted a study involving tens of thousands of people; it concluded that those who slept less than 6? hours or more than 12? hours are significantly more vulnerable to cancer and other diseases than those whose sleep falls into the average range.

Excessive sleep not only can cause physical illness and other dysfunctions but is a primary symptom and manifestation of depression. One of the fundamental objectives of my work and writing is to ensure that you get adequate restful sleep.

Preparatory contemplation, meditation or prayer is the best way to ensure sound sleep. If necessary, you might also utilize safe herbs to help you. If neither is successful, temporary use of pharmaceuticals prescribed by an allopathic practitioner is a viable but undesirable option.

It took me many years of work with many thousands of people to conclude that even pharmaceuticals are preferable to the effects of lost sleep. Not only does chronic sleep deprivation interfere with your life and waste your energy, it often leads to immunological dysfunction and premature death.

Dr. William C. Dement is sleep's foremost authority and the founder of the Sleep Disorder Association. A professor at Stanford University, Dr. Dement recommends trying complementary solutions before resorting to sleep-assisting pharmaceuticals. For example, he suggests such methods as brain acupuncture, a process by which researchers monitor neuronal activity in various parts of the brain in order to discover the best ways to achieve relaxation, rest and sleep, although he indicates that sufficient scientific protocol has not yet been established to validate any long-term efficacy of this process.

He also discusses biofeedback, a technique that allows patients to learn to regulate and control their psychological activities. In this process, machines monitor the brain waves of participants; information provided by the machine allows them to control tension and improve relaxation. Research indicates that biofeedback can be effective but needs machinery to implement it. And he mentions hypnosis as a possible procedure to benefit the sleep-deprived. He says that hypnosis relieves people of undue anxiety, one of the prime causes of sleeplessness, and supports the idea of self-hypnosis, a technique similar in both implementation and effect to meditation. He cites a study in which participants were instructed to lie still, close their eyes, and think of the words "in" and "out" in conjunction with inhalation and exhalation until they fell asleep. Results revealed that this practice is as effective at fighting insomnia as other relaxation techniques.

Dr. Dement insists that we do have various legitimate ways to combat impediments to consistent, full, satisfying and energizing sleep, but adds that sleep problems must be addressed immediately, before they become increasingly severe.

Research and practical wisdom indicate that sleep loss is an incremental process that becomes worse if it is not stopped. However, proper consistent implementation of The Longevity Program has been overwhelmingly effective in combating all sleep disorders. The Program also reduces initial sleep interference and lessens established sleep deprivation.

In his book *Lights Out*, T. S. Wiley writes that sleep disorders began with the availability of artificial light. Until relatively recently, our sleep cycles followed the processes of nature: We functioned during daylight and rested at night. However, our schedules and accompanying metabolism changed after technology made it possible to see at night, and affected in these wholesale changes were such fundamental aspects of daily life as diet, work, exercise, recreation and travel. After many years of altered metabolism, changes in brain chemistry were inevitable. These changes generated a cerebral sensitivity that engenders sleep impediment, including severe sleep deprivation.

The amount and the quality of our rest — especially of our sleep — determine the strength of our immune system and the efficacy of our red blood cells. International studies verify the desire, efforts and success of flourishing seniors to guarantee and protect their sleep. Obviously, healthy patterns of sleep are critical to sustaining functional and fulfilling longevity.

OTHER IMPORTANT FORMS OF REST

Although sleep is our most important form of rest, it must be supported by other forms of rest as well: naps, contemplation/mediation/prayer, communing with nature, harmonious interaction with oneself and others (including non-humans), music, massage, saunas, steam baths, whirlpools, acupressure, acupuncture, chi quing, tai chi, and, along with proper living, the establishment of inner peace. Other restful and fulfilling practices include environmental aesthetics such as feng shui and ikebana (flower arranging), reading, art including painting, photography and sculpture, drama, dance, and music both vocal and instrumental. These positive activities remove us from our routine, allowing us to celebrate ourselves and our best endeavors, and, by accomplishing them we not only relax and rest but we also fulfill and amplify ourselves and our world.

Restful activity — including sleep — moves our brain into the alpha state that is the haven of rest and calm. Like great music, the harmonious rhythm of life cannot be served without the necessary rests, so play the symphony of longevity and enjoy the harmony.

CHAPTER EIGHT

PRACTICAL PROGRESS: DAILY SUGGESTIONS FOR YOUR REJUVENATING JOURNEY

For more than fifty years, we have worked with people at various levels of health from many nations, helping them refine their daily activities, increase their productivity, maximize their creativity, and extend their longevity. In this chapter, we offer a generalized daily plan for enriched and enriching longevity. You have great latitude in your choices; however, all regular routines must include proper diet, appropriate exercise, constant contemplation, sufficient rest and universally beneficial activity. Please proceed at your own pace, but reevaluate that pace frequently to plan and perfect your progress. (A suggested plan for daily dietary implementation of The Longevity Program is provided in Chapter Four.)

WAKING

When you awaken from restful sleep, your positive life will automatically channel your thoughts to the fulfilled, happy, productive life you have created. This is the foundation of the passionate day that will be filled with all of your successes — personal, familial, professional, recreational and universal.

If you are sufficiently fortunate to awaken with a loving companion beside you, glory in that fact and let it propel your passion to fulfill your day.

Look around your peaceful room to appreciate the environmental harmony that you have created through your affirmative life. You do not revel in your materialistic surroundings, but in the fact that these surroundings represent the person whom you are becoming.

LIQUID NOURISHMENT AND NATURAL ELIMINATION

Once you have embraced the unity of everyone and everything around you, proceed to serve your naturally functioning internal harmony. Drink plenty of such healthy liquids as pure water, vegetable and sprout juice, diluted organic fruit juice, herbal tea, fresh grain grass juice, etc. These invigorating fluids will re-hydrate your brain/body and assist healthy eliminatory processes. This step is essential for your body to function at its best throughout the day, because unrestricted circulation of your bloodstream fuels your organs with the oxygen and nutrients necessary for building and repairing the anatomy. Pure blood must permeate the brain barrier, promoting and supporting its maximal functioning, a functioning that is critical to the consistently optimal performance of the entire system.

NATURAL SUPPLEMENTATION: WHOLE FOOD VITAMIN/MINERAL, HERBAL, AND HOMEOPATHIC

In order to defeat the devastating impact of free radical damage (the cause of all aging and disease), malnutrition (the degeneration of the cells and organs of the body), and protein deficiency (insufficiency of amino acids), you must provide your body with adequate healthy supplementation. We derive most of our supplemental nutrients from The Longevity Diet. But to achieve maximal vitality we must add to our diet nutrients that provide protection, purpose and power.

While each individual has unique nutritional needs, universal nutritional requirements are applicable to the great majority of us; here is a list of supplements that serve longevity:

WHOLE FOOD SUPPLEMENTATION:

Vitamins, minerals, enzymes, and their non-cooked derivatives. The Hippocrates Life Extension Supplement Plan includes the following nutrients, all of which should preferably be consumed every morning of every day. (*Please consult an experienced, knowledgeable, sympathetic practitioner in instances of illness or other systematic distress*).

A. Blue-green algae for the brain/body: Take two capsules or 1/4 dropper.

B. Digestive enzymes to combat free radicals and assist digestion: Take four to six capsules before each meal of solid food.

C. Alpha-lipoic acid: 200 milligrams per day.

D. CoQ10: 100 to 200 milligrams.

E. Whole food vitamin C: 100 milligrams per day.

F. For women only: Gota kola: 100 to 200 milligrams.

G. For men only: Pure ginseng: 100 to 200 milligrams.

A study by the European researcher, Dr. Eduard Giovannucci indicates that viruses flourish in a body that lacks nutrition, colds thrive in an anatomy that is deficient in selenium and vitamin C, and Parkinson's disease becomes more likely and more intense in a person who lacks CoQ10.

REST

Every day must include periods of regular rest, if possible, as well as a good night's sleep. When it comes to rest, we should take our cue from non-human creatures, all of whom rest whenever necessary unless they are faced with exceptional circumstances. Although modern life makes regular daily rest difficult for many people, we must create situations that allow us as much of this life-giving and longevity-promoting resource as possible.

SLEEP: THE ULTIMATE REST

Throughout this work and others we tout the critical importance of proper sleep. Every adult should sleep from 8 to 81/2 hours a night, without interruption; children need even more. You must do everything possible to provide you and your family with the availability of restful nightly slumber.

The legs of the tripod that supports your functional longevity are whole-food supplements and proper rest, including sleep. This foundation guarantees vigor, resilience, success, and fulfilling continuity. Do not deny yourself any of these legs; instead, make each of them as strong as possible from day to day.

CHAPTER NINE

COME TO YOUR SENSES
AND LET THEM COME TO YOU

Our use and enjoyment of our senses should not alter merely because of the incursions of age. Our senses connect us with and to the greater world outside ourselves, thus allowing us to appreciate both it and ourselves. In this chapter, we shall discuss how you can maximize both the use and enjoyment of your five senses.

SIGHT

Even if you live to be a thousand, you will never come close to seeing all the wonders of this wonderful world. Vision is the venue to such magnificent natural and man-made wonders as the Seven Wonders of the World, the pyramids, Machu Pichu, the Eiffel Tower, the Great Wall of China, King Tut's tomb, the Taj Mahal, the Rocky Mountains and rain forests. It is no accident that the synonymous phrase for "I understand" is "I see." So it is obvious that we must care for our eyes; in fact, our eyes are so critical that we must care for everyone's eyes by not creating pollution and other blights on our sight.

The nutrients in raw green vegetables such as the antioxidants lutein and zeaxanthin protect and strengthen the tissues of the eyes, improving and increasing vision. *Scientific Daily* reported a study conducted by Professor Joshua Bomser at Ohio State University in which the professor and his colleagues concluded that UV-induced eye damage is reduced by as much as 60 percent when these two vital nutrients are regular parts of a diet.

It is imperative that we protect our eyes at all times; in order to do this, we must wear sunglasses, goggles and all kinds of eye protection.

International studies have proven that exposure to constant powerful sunlight causes twice as many cataracts as protection from it. And it is equally critical that we not strain our eyes by trying to read without glasses if those glasses are necessary. In conjunction with our possible need for glasses and general eye care, we should have our eyes examined by a sympathetic practitioner on a regular basis.

HEARING

Our hearing enriches us, entertains us, and protects us: From the gurgling of a baby to the sound of flowing water to the wailing sirens of emergency vehicles, our ears provide access to emotions and experiences that give our lives dimension and breadth. Unfortunately, one of the plagues of modern life is constant, unpleasant, destructive noise. We must insulate our delicate ears from these offenses as much as possible: Use ear plugs when necessary, enjoy the silence of contemplation, revel in the calming sounds of nature, and keep ears clean at all times — externally and internally — without damaging them. As with our eyes, our ears must be regularly examined by a qualified practitioner.

SMELL

Odors, whether fragrant or foul, please, provoke, protect, pacify, purify, and pollute us. Our sense of smell has become increasingly important in this age of pleasant vapors and hideous pollution. Aromatherapy is among the most compelling examples of the intense effect aromas have on our entire being. Many stimuli of both brain and body — from septic to antiseptic — enter through our nasal passages. Research by Professor Tim Jacob of Cardiff University reported in the journal of the American College of Neuropsychopharmacology reveals that the sense of smell is more acute before meals than after because the chemistry of the brain and body is altered as a result of eating. At Columbia University, Dr. Davangere Devian and his colleagues conducted a study of Alzheimer's disease, testing the effect of 150 scents on participants who suffered from minimal to mild cognitive impairment. Their research proved that those who could not identify the smells of lemon, lilac, heather, clove, menthol, pineapple, natural gas, soap, and strawberries often developed Alzheimer's disease. The results of this investigation support the scientifically established fact that one of the primary symptoms of dementia is the loss of the sense of smell. So not only is a sense of smell important to health and well-being, its unnecessary degeneration is a basis for scientific and medical investigation and consequent correction of various forms of dementia. However, do not assume that all nasal problems indicate degeneration of mental faculties or that all such degeneration is detectable by olfactory testing.

TASTE

Our sense of taste is a developmental process. Imagine our ancestors experimenting with various tastes for the first time, trying everything from succulent fruits to inedible bitters. Taste provokes, stimulates and generates everything from the physical to the figurative, including memory, digestive enzymes, habits and patterns both good and bad, and diet (both nutritious and addictive). We must refine our sense of taste to make it consistent with our overall development. It is no accident that the phrase "to have good taste" refers to a person's general sense of discernment.

The receptor cells of our taste buds send clear messages to every part of the body and brain. An unpleasant flavor can affect the entire nervous system so severely that it causes the body to shake as it disgorges that violator. On the other hand, a savory delight may also course through the body, fulfilling it far beyond the merely physical. So we must always try to select that which is "taste-full," and consume only that which is healthy, knowing that what we taste eventually affects our entire health — including our longevity.

TOUCH

Among our remarkable senses, touch is the one that connects us most intimately to and with the physical world. By touch, we do not mean only that which is touched by our hands and feet; touch also means that which touches our bodies in any way, good or bad — from the warmth of the sun to the pain of an open flame. It is no accident that the expression "profoundly touched" indicates the effect of a compelling phenomenon on the total person. To be profoundly touched is to feel the most intense perception, sympathy, empathy, harmony and love.

Research at the University of Miami's Touch Therapy Center indicates that the immune systems of infants who are consistently and lovingly touched in therapeutic and appropriate ways function at maximum levels, affording them the best health and the strongest resistance to disease and distress. These benefits apply to people of all ages, including those enjoying their maturity.

Since touch is so intimate and important, each of us must touch others only lovingly, positively and beneficially. As Tim Rice wrote for the Andrew Lloyd Webber musical *Cats*,

> *Touch me;*
> *it's so easy to leave me*
> *all alone with my memory*
> *of my days in the sun.*
> *If you touch me,*
> *you'll understand what happiness is.*
> *Look —*
> *a new day has begun.*

COMMON SENSE

The anecdotal "sixth sense" is, in fact, extremely real: It is common sense, which is not at all common but, rather, extremely rare. Ironically, it is called "common" because it is something all sentient beings should have "in common." As we noted with our other senses, the application of language is again appropriately descriptive, because "feeling" people are those who "feel" — touched emotionally so profoundly that the experience penetrates their cores.

"Common sense" is the combination of intellect, insight, intuition and instinct, and, since this is the case, progressive longevity enhances common sense and facilitates its application to daily life.

CHAPTER 10

PRESERVE PASSION

Let us discuss the preservation of passion naturally, physically, and intellectually; in the next chapter, we can discuss the imperative preservation and promotion of romance.

Passion is defined as an "intense feeling," but that intensity of feeling must be channeled positively to constitute authentic passion. Distortions of passion such as violence and other illogical behavior are merely violations of passion. We must reverse this negative inclination and infuse our best with all "passionate intensity."

If you live in a way that is positively impassioned, you benefit yourself, your immediate environment, and all of life. This capacity is also intensified through constructive longevity.

PURE PASSION PROLONGS LIFE

Recall the unbridled intensity of childhood: As children, we run freely, sing spontaneously, dance uninhibitedly, interact innocently, and love unrestrictedly. Then, as time and influences impose themselves upon us, we are restrained and constrained by limitations that may remain with us through life, inhibiting not only longevity but also healthy functioning at every age.

Many people recollect their youth ruefully in two mutually ironic ways: They would love to rectify their mistakes, but they would also be happy to return to it because they feel trapped by the aging process. The most satisfying solution is to enjoy the best of both worlds: Retain the vitality of youth, buttressed by the wisdom of maturity. Both processes require positive passion. In order to sustain the vitality of youth, you must unburden yourself of those problems and concerns that are injurious to you and irrelevant to youth. You must act courageously to choose what is ultimately best for you and dismiss whatever might appear to provide short-term benefits but in fact imposes long-term stress and distress.

The most important contribution you can make to your longevity is to live an impassioned life; those who love what they do love how they live. Positive passion is the best way to prolong your path and flourish freely.

INTENSE PASSION INTENSIFIES LIFE

If you recall the times in your life when you were intensely involved in an exciting project and floating on a cloud of concentrated creativity, you may remember how quickly the time passed even when it seemed to last forever. Our greatest contributors, passionate people who devoted their essences to their passions and donated their intensity to universal benefit, have all either sustained positive longevity or expended themselves gloriously in their commitment.

If we work together in positive concert, this self-directed passion will dispel all problems and energize the environment.

PURPOSEFUL PASSION
KEEPS YOU IN YOUR PRIME

Focused commitment to, and implementation of, your positive passions allows you the power to proceed progressively. If you expand your needs in concert with nature, you will also serve nature in concert with your needs. Purpose in your life adds power to your longevity, but you must identify, implement and intensify that purpose: Without it, you will remain unfulfilled and incomplete. The road to healthy longevity commences at commitment, continues through determination, and concludes at achievement. As you expand your positive, purposeful life to include family, friends, community, environment and entirety, you fulfill and strengthen both yourself and the passion with which you started.

PASSION SUPPORTS PROPRIETY
AND PROPRIETY ILLUMINATES PASSION

The charming French word "etiquette" supplies a surprising aspect of passion. At first it might appear that propriety and civility are distant from passion; however, a well-lived life encourages and promotes the kind of harmonious interaction with life that is the manifestation of etiquette. We must be as intense in our commitment to suitable behavior as we are to all other life-serving functions. Proper behavior enhances self-respect, allowing us to fulfill our objectives and embrace the successful life that serves ourselves and our lives.

PASSIONATE PROSPERITY

Work is a necessary and positive aspect of life. You can prosper in every way if you love what you do by doing what you love. The rewards of work beyond the financial are many: Satisfaction; fulfillment; positive productivity; self improvement; harmonious relationships; universal enrichment; the satisfaction of contribution; a legacy of integrity. Best of all, the benefits of work can fuel your passion.

Because fulfilling work is so essential to our lives, lack of satisfaction with our work often causes a domino effect that leads to the disintegration of other aspects of life. We need to stop this destructive process at the beginning: If you do not like your work — for whatever reason — choose among those occupations that provide you with rewards beyond the merely monetary.

You can reeducate yourself and train for whatever profession inspires that passion — so whatever your work is to be, make sure it serves the greater sphere as it rewards you.

CREATIVE RECREATION

The cooperative partner of work is play. We must have recreation that engages our passions and promotes our lives. Work without play and play without work are both unsatisfactory; we need play to liberate us from the structure of work, and work to create the structure for our recreation.

Exhilarating hobbies are, in their own way, as inspiring as invigorating work.

Among the most rewarding of many physical diversions are gardening, dancing, walking, swimming, diving, aerobic exercise and resistance exercise, skiing, surfing, sailing, windsailing, Ping-Pong (table tennis) and lovemaking (about which we write more in the next chapter). We also have many more leisurely hobbies: painting, pottery, singing, board games, billiards, croquet and, again, lovemaking.

We can also fulfill ourselves recreationally by enjoying many cultural pursuits, among which are enjoying painting, sculpture and architecture in both museums and outdoors; attending plays, ballet, concerts of all varieties from classical to country, or poetry and prose readings. Once you have indulged such favorites, it is time for the passion that should be indulged day or night, young or old: Romance. (Please proceed passionately to the following chapter.)

CHAPTER ELEVEN

REJOICE: RETAIN — AND REINVIGORATE — ROMANCE

"Grandpa Bill is on the hill with someone he just married;
there he is at 93, doing what comes naturally!"
(Irving Berlin in *Annie Get Your Gun*)

For the wise, romance is in everything; for the mature, romance is everywhere. It is not only the beloved, but what is provided by nature, art, achievement and serenity. Experience intensifies our appreciation of intimacy.

In Shakespeare's *Antony and Cleopatra*, Mark Antony says of Cleopatra, "Age cannot wither her, nor custom stale her infinite variety." A significant part of the romance of life involves the romance between loving partners. The passionate intimacy of romantic love is limited by nothing, certainly not time: Live well, and you will love well.

Joan and Stephen Wagner had been married for 62 years when they attended The Institute. Each had serious disorders at the time: Stephen came to us from a hospital where his condition had been misdiagnosed and his treatment mismanaged to the brink of death; Joan had been told that arthritis would cripple her and that she had signs of dementia. During their brief stay with us and thereafter, their health was reinvigorated. As part of the consultation process, I asked them what had been the most frightening aspect of their pre-Hippocrates experience. Almost immediately and in unison, they replied that it was their loss of intimacy, which they feared was permanent. I asked about the frequency of their intimacy, and this 80-plus couple again responded simultaneously: "At least five times a week."

At first I was amazed by this revelation; but when I thought about it, I realized that, although they might have been statistical anomalies, in fact they should be the norm. In fact, they are the norm for many seniors in Asia, whose romantic potency is sustained throughout their lives. Why is this so?

The answer involves the many positive aspects of Asian longevity that are often missing from the lives of people on other continents; focused and disciplined minds and a healthy mode of living, including vegetarian food and excluding obesity. Asian cultures have retained the respect for maturity that is severely lacking in much of the rest of the world, and this self-maintained and self-activated respect fuels the passion and vitality that invigorate sexual longevity.

THE PHYSICAL AND PSYCHOLOGICAL BENEFITS OF LOVEMAKING

Lovemaking, historically the source of the greatest joy, unifies two loving souls into one loving entity. Of the many glories bestowed upon us by nature and ourselves, none supersedes the intense, comprehensive, profound glory of lovemaking.

Science validates our appreciation of this unique phenomenon; research has proven that the exceptional elevation of hormonal levels produced by making love suffuses the brain with positive chemistries that negate depression and activate and intensify the immune system. One's generation of orgasmic secretions requires magnified utilization of leukocytes (white blood cells), allowing us to feel fulfilled and relaxed during and after this sublime experience.

Intimacy involves more than sex: In fact, true intimacy requires the manifestation of many other aspects of an intimate romantic relationship, including respect, affection, companionship, caring, cuddling, and sharing the entirety of the life experience.

Scientific studies involving breast and prostate cancer prove that consistent healthy sexual activity can actually diminish the intensity, the likelihood or the existence of these serious health problems. Our entire hormonal system — including pheromones, the secretions that emit engaging erotic scents — needs constant reinvigoration in order to renew biochemical balance. Because the commitment and durability of lifelong romance unify loving couples, the loss of a lover is devastating, particularly after many years together. Once the initial mourning period has passed, however, begin focusing on the profound beauty and indelible memory of your union.

Because lovemaking is an essential element of adult functioning, lengthy abstinence — whether chosen or situational — depletes the strength of the body and the resilience of the emotions.

Historically, prohibitions against sexual intimacy have existed in many societies around the globe. We can ascribe these impositions to those who established these societies; they constructed rigid social systems at the expense of individual fulfillment. Although these people sought to eliminate or minimize the socially undesirable consequences of certain unions, they ignored or dismissed the value of the intimacy they were attempting to inhibit.

While masturbation is an adequate form of release, it does not replicate either the emotional or the physical benefits and rewards of lovemaking. Monogamous sexual intimacy fuels the fire of life, heats the soul and warms the heart; it also circulates the balanced temperature of fulfillment throughout the self.

Unfortunately, we are plagued by problems that inhibit this celebration of our bodies, especially as we age. It is estimated that one-third of the male population in so-called "Western" countries and one-quarter of its female population have difficulties with intimacy, fulfillment and procreation. These problems can generally be attributed to the excessive consumption of meat and dairy products, which inhibit the flow of blood and oxygen and reduce both sexual desire and sexual activity. Meat and dairy are toxic agents that also cause weight gain, obesity, clogged arteries, malaise, generally declining health and excessively rapid aging.

Researchers at Duke University have determined that approximately 80 percent of American males in their late 60s continue to be sexually active while only 25 percent of American men in their late 70s and older continue sexual activity. Additional research reveals that only 60 percent of American men in their early 40s manifest sexual initiative and stamina. These alarming statistics indicate that sedentary and stressful modern lifestyles are depleting these men of their potency — not only sexually but also personally, professionally, creatively and recreationally. Also, as many as 60 percent of the women in these societies admit to faking orgasms, not only to placate their partners but to disguise the lack of vaginal sensitivity that deprives them of orgasms.

Sexual problems are rampant among the mature inhabitants of "Western" nations, where older men suffer not only from an alarming rate of sexual dysfunction but also from maladies of the prostate.

The extraordinary joy of lovemaking, which we discover in our youth and enjoy during our lives, should accompany us throughout maturity: The fact that it often does not means we have sabotaged one of our greatest gifts, and that in order to have a fulfilling longevity — "the last of life for which the first of life was made," wrote poet Robert Browning — we must reclaim romance.

NOURISHING APHRODISIACS

"If music be the food of love, play on," writes Shakespeare at the beginning of *Twelfth Night*. While music might set the mood for love, there is ample "food of love." Among the best aphrodisiacal sources (to be taken individually and sparingly, as recommended) are these:

APRICOTS; APRICOT SEEDS: Apricots and their seeds contain abscisic acid (B-17), a cancer-preventing substance that activates, invigorates and sustains sexual hormones. Consumption of apricots does not provide the comprehensive benefits provided by their seeds, so you should have 5 to 15 apricot seeds several hours before any anticipated intimacy.

BLACK RASPBERRY (FRUIT AND SEEDS): This brain stimulating phytochemical-rich food enhances libido and endurance. Black-raspberry seeds contain plenty of nourishment to fuel intimacy. Have 10 black raspberries or, preferably, one tablespoon or soup spoon of the seeds two hours before anticipated intimacy.

DILL: This exceptionally nutritious herb is of particular benefit to women because of its ability to increase both the number and the structure of eggs. It also enhances the desire for intimacy. Take sunflower green sprouts — 7.5 milliliters (1/2 ounce) — before intercourse.

FIGS: Fresh figs contain nutrients that are considered excellent stimulants of fertility. They also enhance the secretion of pheromones, maximizing physical appeal. Eat three to five figs when you and your partner are sexually in the mood.

FLOWER POLLEN: The consumption of this pollen increases the number of leukocytes (white blood cells), strengthening the body for erotic adventure. Have one tablespoon or soup spoon of it every morning because, in addition to its aphrodisiacal qualities, flower pollen is an almost complete food that provides exceptional nutrition.

HIBISCUS: The fine sun tea from this flower is delightful to sip before, during and after intimacy, because it stimulates the glands involved in sexual activity.

JERUSALEM ARTICHOKE: This root vegetable, which is derived from the sunflower family, contains a unique form of complex carbohydrates that provides fortified energy without the sugars that attack the pancreas. The energy of Jerusalem artichokes invigorates the life force both generally and sexually. Consume 120 milliliters (four ounces) during the morning of the day's anticipated intimacy.

LENTIL SPROUTS: The minerals and vitamins in these sprouts increase the cellular activity of the sexually inciting hormones. Have 90 to 150 milliliters (three to five ounces) one hour before intimacy.

LETTUCE: Lettuce — especially iceberg lettuce — contains an opiate that activates sex hormones; as a result, it has been a popular aphrodisiac for millennia. Consume one bowlful approximately three hours before intimacy.

MULBERRIES: These phytonutrient-rich fruits are a historically validated aphrodisiac that couples have enjoyed as a source of seduction. Eat one or two handfuls just before foreplay.

NUTMEG: This aphrodisiacal herb literally heats the ovaries, fueling a woman's sexual desire. Have three or four milliliters (2 1/8 ounces) one hour before any anticipated intimacy.

OAT SPROUTS: "Sow your wild oats" is not merely a colloquial expression, but a figurative representation of the beginning of an established aphrodisiacal practice. Consuming oat sprouts in their pure form increases the production of eggs and sperm, infusing you with sexual vitality. Take 90 to 120 milliliters (three to four ounces) three to four hours before probable intimacy.

PEA GREENS: This protein-rich sprout contains significant concentrations of amino acids to enhance the production of red blood cells, thereby causing sexual arousal in males. Juice and drink 60 to 120 milliliters (two to four ounces) an hour before intimacy. Eating pea greens in salad form also provides modest erotic stimulation.

RADICCHIO: This leafy vegetable furnishes minerals and trace minerals that encourage and enhance sexual endurance in both women and men. Have 1/11th liter (two ounces) eight hours before anticipated intimacy.

SPELT SPROUTS: The combination of vitamins and amino acids in these protein-rich grains increases sexual endurance by increasing healthy hormone count. Eat one cup two to four hours before intimacy.

TOMATO SEEDS (ONLY ORGANIC): The seeds of sun-dried organic tomatoes contain various phytonutrients that invigorate glands and promote the development of sex hormones. Have 1/11th to 1/7th liters (two to three ounces) an hour before intimacy.

WATERMELON SEED SPROUTS: The condensed complete proteins in these sprouts increase the number of leukocytes (white blood cells), thereby enhancing general vitality and sensual intensity. Juice and drink 180 milliliters (six ounces) four hours before intimate activity.

YAMS: Raw yams — either grated or sprouted — elevate hormonal levels (including those of estrogen, progesterone, testosterone, DHEA, DHA, etc.) of both women and men, preparing and prompting each to perform effectively and at length. Consume 1/7th to 1/3rd liters (three to six ounces) two hours before contact.

ZUCCHINI (raw or juiced): The deep roots of this summer squash absorb trace minerals that build both red and white blood cells, helping to cleanse veins and capillaries, enhancing the circulation of oxygen that increases and intensifies both desire and performance. Eat either an entire zucchini (two to three ounces) or drink 60 to 90 milliliters (again, two to three ounces) three hours before each performance . . . and don't be surprised by an encore!

The combination of romantic love, exhilarating thought, and nutritional enhancement elevates erotic pleasure to sublime exhilaration; enjoy every minute of it.

CHAPTER TWELVE

LIBERATED LIVING:
FREE YOURSELF FROM STRESS

Ironically, the apparent progress of modern life continues to impose increased stress on all of us. Schedules — work, family, transportation and every other imposed form of relaxation and recreation — dominate our world and create more stress on us than ever. Since this is the case, we must seek to liberate ourselves from stress-inducing stimuli.

Stress has always been a major cause of premature aging; contemporary science has proven this. Drs. Elissa Epel and Elizabeth Blackburn of the University of California, San Francisco led a team of researchers that analyzed the blood samples of young and middle-aged mothers who care for children with such chronic disorders as autism and cerebral palsy. As part of their genetic technique evaluations, these scientists studied the DNA of the participants' white blood cells because that DNA is essential to the body's immune response to infection. They focused on the part of the DNA called the telomere, which rests at the tip of each cell's chromosome as prominently as the head on a matchstick. The telomere strikes each time a cell divides or replicates itself. Cells can reproduce themselves many times in order to strengthen their host organs, allowing the organs to regenerate, grow, strengthen and fight disease. A chemical, telomeres, helps restore a portion of the telomere after each division.

After 10 to 50 divisions, the telomere becomes so short that the cell is too fatigued to regenerate. Those who are born with the genetic disease dyskeratosis congenita, which causes accelerated curtailment of telomeres, generally die in middle age because of compromised immunity. The chronological changes of the length of a telomere might indicate the level of a cell's age and vitality. When they compared the DNA of the stress-imposed mothers caring for their disabled children to the DNA of the victims of dyskeratosis congenita, the researchers discovered that the increasing duration of stressful care causes the degeneration (and diminishing length) of telomeres, drastically accelerating the aging process. Many of the tested mothers were determined — by scientific evaluation of their white blood cells — to be much older physically than they were in comparison to their chronological ages. These discoveries magnified the absolute connection between chronic psychological stress and weakened immune function.

Many factors determine an individual's response to stress. A compelling study from New Zealand has demonstrated that we are born with genetic protection from stress. When the self-protective anti-stress genes are compromised, we are vulnerable to greater amounts and intensities of stress. The researchers evaluated people from birth to the age of 26; they were able to predict which of the participants would become susceptible to depression caused by personal calamities such as divorce and unemployment.

FIGHT MIDAFTERNOON MALAISE

Most of us ingest sugar, caffeine or cake to elevate our systems from the semi-coma of mid-afternoon. Why is midday so demanding, and why does it make us so restless? Perhaps it's simply sleep deprivation caused by demanding schedules. Dr. Bob Strickgold, Professor of Psychiatry at Harvard Medical School, has said that man is the only organism that deprives itself of sleep. The constitution of most mammals allows them to stay awake after intense and rapidly changing emotional stimuli. Monkeys and many other creatures observe their natural need for rest before any social or societal impetus. Unfortunately, our modern 9-to-5 world does not accommodate human metabolism, and, ironically, our inability to rest at midday interferes with nightly sleep as well as with our daily activities. Historically, humans rested at mid-afternoon, as shown by the practice of the siesta throughout many parts of the world. Many noted colleagues, most of whom achieved healthy and productive longevity, have been practicing advocates of midday rest, including architect Buckminster Fuller, scientists Thomas Edison and Albert Einstein and humanitarian Albert Schweitzer.

Researchers have discovered that most subjects who eat regularly but have no access to any time-measuring devices, tend to fall asleep during two parts of a day — at 1-4 A.M. and 1-4 P.M. It is during these periods that our Circadian rhythms are their highest pitch and body temperatures are elevated, inducing sleep, so both science and the human systems that it measures indicate that we are intended to sleep four hours of every twelve rather than eight of every 24.

As we have learned from the sleepiness that follows eating, we are also subject to a postprandial dip after every meal. Dr. Sara Mednick, a researcher at the Salk Institute, has said that these sleep inducements often occur even when eating has not preceded them. She maintains that the desire to return to sleep is present from the moment we awake, and believes that during the Middle Ages people napped regularly. However, the advent of timepieces, light-bulbs, factories and commuting to work have made this natural inclination impossible for most of us. The development of modern life has also created a need for many of us to work at night, during the conventional natural sleep cycle, causing not only stress but also vulnerability to disease and impaired longevity. All of this is additional evidence that our regular need for restful sleep is based on a 12-hour — not a 24-hour — cycle.

If we must sleep on the 24-hour cycle, we need to ensure that our sleep is not interrupted. Segments of sleep interrupted by stretches of waking undermine all physical activity as well as restricting thought and hindering longevity. Research conducted by Dr. Edward Stepanoski of Rush University Medical Center has proven that the uncomfortable and unhealthy pattern of dozing and waking causes alterations of natural brain-wave patterns. A modest amount of noise or a disturbing dream — even your own body movement — can impede the quality and security of sleep.

Because lack of sleep causes other problems, we must combat both that lack and the problems it causes, one of which is unwanted weight gain. Dr. Steven Heymsfield of Columbia University and St. Luke's Roosevelt Hospital maintains that it is possible to help people sleep better and longer while simultaneously helping them regulate their weight.

Dr. Heymsfield and Dr. James Gangwisch, epidemiologist at Columbia University, conducted an extensive 10-year study of the lives and habits — good and bad — of 18,000 adults to determine the connection between nutrition and sleep. Their initial notion was that increased sleep caused obesity because the activity that expends the fewest calories is rest. Instead, they discovered to their amazement, one of our foremost activities when we are awake is eating, and much of what we eat not only decreases health but also increases weight. This overeating causes chronic sleep deprivation because the circuitry of the body/brain becomes wired for periods of gorging food instead of seeking rest.

As a result of this and other studies, many scientists and medical practitioners have concluded that lack of sleep, overeating and weight gain are a vicious, life-depleting cycle. Dr. Heymsfield has said that there is a convincing body of scientific evidence proving the connection among sleep patterns, eating patterns, weight problems and malnutrition.

"Not all sleep is created equal" is an axiom of sleep researchers, because each night's sleep is segmented into five constantly altering stages that can be measured by the types of brain waves that reflect the depth of one's sleep at any given time. Toward morning, Rapid Eye Movement (REM) increases because our muscles are relaxed, dreaming occurs, and recent memories impose themselves upon our semi-conscious state. Compromised sleep during this crucial period may precipitate distress and dysfunction during the following day, and the accumulation of disturbed sleep has such permanent consequences as the premature aging that leads to a shortened lifespan.

Dr. Arthur Spielman, Professor of Psychology and Sleep researcher at City College of the City University of New York, cites many studies that have proven that sleep impairment also impairs memory, reaction time, comprehension, attention span and even emotional balance. He says that the first indications of sleep deprivation are usually extreme irritability and increasing depression, causing stress both to the sleep-deprived individual and those around him. These symptoms are obvious results of the loss of the necessary rest that keeps us centered.

Dr. Spielman says this about continual loss of sleep: "Creativity and zest for life are dampened. You just don't feel like doing much. However, there is a growing realization that chronic sleep loss affects health, from minor disturbances like headaches to an increased risk for obesity, diabetes and cardiovascular disease."

Clearly, in the vicious cycle that is stress, all of these maladies are both caused by stress and cause stress themselves.

How can we fight this scourge? Encouraging research indicates that we can combat lost sleep with meditation, contemplation, prayer, yoga, regular exercise, soothing music, reduced stress, harmonious interaction, and romantic intimacy. We must also refrain from eating or drinking anything for at least two hours before we go to sleep for the night.

Healthy longevity requires a combination of contributing factors; among the most important of these is complete regular rest, especially sleep. The Longevity Program includes techniques that foster relaxation and promote the deeply restful sleep that diminishes stress and intensifies creativity. If your sleep is profound, you become profound. If your sleep is complete, you become complete. If you provide yourself with liberal sleep, you will liberate your sleep from deficiency and yourself from a great deal of stress.

CHAPTER THIRTEEN

NATURAL HEALTH. . . NATURALLY

If we approach our longevity naturally, our problems are few. Although maturity has its own problems, you can probably deal with them at home. Here are some concerns often associated with advanced aging, even though they occur at every age, and what you can do about them:

ADDICTION

We cannot confuse choice with compulsion, so we must be strong enough to choose and never become weak enough to submit. The many addictive behaviors of our time are among our most distressing, life-draining and longevity-inhibiting problems. The list of addiction-causing substances is long and singularly undistinguished, including alcohol, tobacco, heroin, cocaine, marijuana, and prescription drugs. Even more prevalent than these scourges is the almost universal addiction to "food." Addiction is caused by lack of self-respect, but if we live fulfilling, rewarding, beneficial lives, we will feel no need to indulge in the abuse of counterproductive substances and behaviors.

GROUP THERAPY: Multi-step anti-addiction programs have proven successful for many participants. This kind of group interaction moves the plagued individual from addictive isolation to the shared universal experience that encourages and aids acceptance of self and dismissal of pathologically self-destructive behavior. Since addictive patterns, whatever the substance, are relatively uniform, legitimate treatment programs to counteract them are also similar.

OTHER THERAPIES: Acupuncture, acupressure, cranial-sacral therapy, shiatsu, watsu (water shiatsu), other appropriate forms of massage and heat therapies help reprogram the brain and body away from addiction and toward affirmative activity.

STABILIZING FOODS: Healthy eating can prevent and neutralize addiction. You must consume food that has plenty of easily digestible protein and little to no cooked carbohydrates. These stabilizing foods include sprouts, sea algae, fresh- water algae, sprouted nuts and seeds, and sprouted mung beans.

OTHER NUTRIENTS: Nori seaweed, wakame seaweed, kava kava, passion flower, hops and parsley have been proven to help combat and allay all forms of addiction.

ALLERGIES

Allergic reactions tend to multiply and intensify for those who mature unhealthily. There exist three basic categories of allergies: those caused by contact; those caused by inhalation of natural, artificial, biological and/or chemical substances; and those caused by "food" (mostly by the kind that is also harmful to consume). Suggested home remedies for each type of allergy follow. Please note that all three types of allergies are airborne — directly by contact and inhalation, and indirectly via "food," especially of the commercial variety. This means that their sources literally travel through the air and settle on all environments, including "food." Until the day comes when we have purged the world of airborne toxins, we must be careful about where we go, what we do, what we eat, what we touch, and with whom we interact in any way.)

A: Contact allergies can be addressed by consistently cleansing and disinfecting your environment, especially your home and workplace. Most important is regular, thorough washing of the face and hands with natural bio-organic solutions. The use of chemicals — including perfume, cologne, cosmetics, toothpaste, soap — is a dangerous and frequent cause of allergic reactions. Another frequent cause of contact allergies is wearing man-made fibers. Physical contact with humans and non-humans is always conducive to many contact allergies.

B: The variety of allergies caused by the air we breathe (and have polluted) has multiplied drastically since the Industrial Revolution. We have produced thousands of substances, most of which can and do cause allergic reactions, some of which can be severe. Modern conveniences such as central heating, central air-conditioning and vacuuming also circulate many allergy-causing particles both man-made and natural, particularly dust mites, molds, fungi, viruses and bacteria.

C: Much of what we eat and drink weakens and destroys both interior and exterior health. "Foods" that cause allergies also weaken every bodily system, increasing the likelihood and severity of premature aging. The most common "food"-based causes of allergies are dairy, meat, and wheat and its derivatives. Some people even manifest allergies to whole natural foods, not because of the foods but because of the chemical imbalance within those people, an imbalance that is, ironically, often caused by their chronic ingestion of meat and dairy.

Here is a list of suggested solutions to combat or eliminate such allergens and the reactions they cause:

AIR FILTRATION — OZONE: (A, B & C): Even the best air filters are ineffective; worse, most collect, breed and disperse the same allergens that they are supposed to combat and eliminate. The Ozone air-purification method is the only viable means of cleansing the atmosphere of our homes and automobiles, our schools, workplaces and other gathering places. These health-promoting units produce oxygen (O3) that actually finds and destroys airborne microbes, carcinogens, biological parasites including dust mites, and other pollutants.

DEHUMIDIFIERS: (A & B): Dehumidifiers reduce humidity by as much as 65 percent, neutralizing the proliferation, mobility and effect of airborne pollutants.

FUNGICIDES: (A, B & C): Your environment and your food should be regularly cleansed by wiping them with natural anti-fungal solutions such as peroxide, which is inexpensive, available, and can be easily diluted with pure water.

WOOD; TILE, MARBLE, AND OTHER NATURAL STONES: (A & B): These natural substances should replace carpeting as environmentally beneficial flooring. Carpets are breeding grounds for pet dander, mites, molds, chemicals, and other dangerous residents. You can, however, place easy-to-clean natural fiber throw rugs on your carpet-free flooring.

FOOD: (C): The exclusively bio-organic Longevity Diet not only provides you with delicious nutrition, but is, with rare exceptions, anti-allergenic. The immunity-building nutrients of The Longevity Menu strengthen the body, allowing it to resist many allergy-causing substances.

HOMEOPATHICS: (A, B & C): This natural pharmacy provides a wide range of allergy-reducing and allergy-eliminating benefits. In addition, homeopathic treatments have neither side effects nor any other counterproductive consequences.

ESSENTIAL OILS: (A & B): Placing essential oils in your nostrils helps relieve allergic reactions and prevent potential ones.

SANITARY MASK: (A & B): During allergy season — and in severely polluted environments — you can temporarily resort to using a sanitary mask, which can be found at medical supply stores because it is used by medical personnel.

ANGINA; HEART DISEASE; STROKE; PHLEBITIS; OTHER CARDIOVASCULAR PROBLEMS

Because these conditions result from unhealthy living, they can be alleviated at home if you change your lifestyle. This requires only two steps:

LIVING VEGETARIAN/VEGAN FOOD(S): Eliminate all animal-based fare from your diet. Consume only raw bio-organic vegan food in order to purify and build your body, increase your immunity, and elevate your health completely, maximizing heart function.

EXERCISE: Exercise consistently and properly, using both aerobics and resistance training. Because the heart is, among other things, a pump, it needs to pump regularly to be at its best.

RELAXATION TECHNIQUES: Forms of reflection, including meditation and prayer, ease the functioning of the chemistry of your entire body, including the brain and the heart. This alleviates and can even prevent cardiovascular concerns. Similar beneficial effects can be realized by communing with nature and art.

NATURAL REMEDIES: Your heart and the rest of the circulatory system are significantly benefited by consumption of raw garlic and garlic-based supplements, capsicum tincture, slippery elm, and herb teas that minimize lipid levels.

ARTHRITIS; RHEUMATISM; RHEUMATOID AND OSTEO ARTHRITIS; RELATED AILMENTS

These problems are among the oldest ailments, so old that anthropologists have discovered that even dinosaurs suffered from them. However, they can be successfully treated at home using the following means:

LIVING VEGETARIAN/VEGAN FOOD(S): The alkaline-producing bounties of living vegetarian/vegan cuisine combat the systematic acidity that is one of the primary causes of rheumatic dysfunctions.

WEIGHT CONTROL and REGULATION: Excess weight makes intense demands on your joints, ligaments, bones, muscles and heart, all of which increase the likelihood and severity of arthritic conditions. In addition, burdensome weight reduces the oxygen content of the blood cells, allowing acidity to dominate the system, which causes pain, brittle bones and the erosion of bone structure and other bodily systems.

WATER EXERCISE: This pleasant form of exercise alleviates gravitational pressure, reducing the pain caused by arthritic conditions. In order to do water exercise, put yourself into chest-deep warm water and wave your arms while walking joyfully in the pool.

HERBAL REMEDIES: White willow bark, valerian, lemon grass and similar herbs can be used to reduce pain and increase flexibility.

ICE PACKS: The application of ice packs to painful joints that have been overworked or are affected by overwork reduces pain and soothes the area.

HEAT PACKS: If your joints become irritated, swollen, hot and/or tender, apply heat packs to them for effective relief.

MASSAGE: These beneficial forms of bodywork replicate the benefits of exercise. Massage facilitates greater circulation, movement and flexibility while reducing pain. Among the many types of effective massage are neuromuscular, shiatsu, Rolfing and structural alignment.

WHOLE-FOOD VITAMIN C: Research conducted at Pennsylvania College of Pediatric Medicine by Dr. Robert H. Davis has proven that those who suffer from rheumatoid arthritis have a serious lack of Vitamin C. The use of sufficient amounts of whole-food Vitamin C in either food or supplement form helps suppress both the commencement and the intensity of these ailments.

EXCLUSIVE CONSUMPTION OF LIVING/RAW FOOD: Eat only fresh, organic, non-cooked vegetarian foods to reconstitute your health and reduce arthritic conditions. Many so called "foods" and other substances aggravate rheumatoid problems and bone degeneration; among the worst are cooked white potatoes, tomatoes, eggplant, peppers (except ripe), and, interestingly, tobacco, all of which are part of the nightshade plant family. Dairy is notorious for complicating these diseases, as are all cooked and fried oils. Raw juices — including those of celery, celeric, cabbage sprouts, broccoli sprouts, onion sprouts, rutabaga, Brussels sprouts, and turnips — help the remission of rheumatoid concerns. Unheated omega oils are most plentiful in hemp and flaxseed; they facilitate recovery from rheumatoid conditions, as proven by the work of Dr. George Blackburn, Chief of Nutrition/Metabolism Laboratory at the Cancer Research Institute of New England.

ASTHMA, (ECZEMA), EMPHYSEMA, AND RELATED CONDITIONS

"Asthma" comes from the Greek phrase "constricted airways." The condition starts with the contraction of the bronchi, which causes tightness of the chest, shortness of breath, coughing and wheezing. More than 90 percent of asthmatics under the age of 40 suffer from allergies to trees, weeds, grass pollens, animal dander, dust mites, pollution and molds. Whatever its cause and its extent, asthma is correctable. Those who suffer from these conditions should avoid extremely cold climates.

FRESH AIR: The best solution is simple, obvious and natural: The best breathing is served by the best air. The problem is that we are destroying our fresh air, making breathing difficult not only for those with breathing problems but for those who never had them. Studies indicate that the air in your home is much more polluted than the air outside it; therefore, leave your windows open slightly whenever possible, especially when you are sleeping. It is also helpful to live in a relatively clean environment rather than in polluted cities. If you must live in a city, give yourself and your family as much time in nature as possible.

OZONE-TREATED AIR: Ordinary air filters are either inadequate or ineffective. Only ozone-treated air actually seeks and completely destroys such pollutants as molds, bacteria, viruses, dust mites, and other microbes. Because ozone kills these toxins, you can breathe more freely inside your home, workplace and vehicle. Systems to circulate ozone-treated air in your home can be purchased worldwide. Wherever you live, avoid smoke-filled environments, indoors and out.

OXYGEN-RICH FOODS: Raw vegetable greens and sprouts, and their juices, contain significant amounts of oxygen to energize the hemoglobin of your red blood cells and reduce both the symptoms and intensity of breathing disorders. Some "foods" induce and aggravate asthma; among the most dangerous are milk, flour, eggs, cooked white potatoes, "seafood" and nuts. Food additives, such as MSG (monosodium glutamate), are even more severe enemies.

To breathe the best, eat foods rich in vitamin B-6 and take whole-food supplements that contain it. Dr. Clayton L. Natta of Columbia University conducted a study in which participants were given megadoses of vitamin B-6. The study revealed that the asthmatic symptoms of these people were reduced significantly as a result.

HERBAL REMEDIES: Consume three to five drops of pure eucalyptus oil in some water or juice twice per day. During one night, put two drops of spearmint or wintergreen on your pillowcase; the next night, use two drops of tea-tree oil. These substances help decongest the cilia of the lungs.

EXERCISE: Healthy exercise of every sort is beneficial to proper breathing. Among the best are walking, swimming and aerobics, all of which allow the lungs to expand and increase their capacity.

BACK PAIN:

Between 30 and 50 percent of "Western" populations suffer from some form of back pain, usually because of improper lifting, bad posture, obesity, too much sitting, inadequate sleep support, accidents, and injuries caused by athletic activity. However, athletic activity that is harmonious with the body is an excellent solution for many back problems.

EXERCISE: Among the best remedies to combat back pain is regulated proper exercise. Two of the best forms of exercise that are not likely to damage your back are walking and swimming; others are dancing, rock climbing, non competitive gymnastics, tai chi and chi quong.

HERBAL REMEDIES: The use of camomile, hops, lobelia and other anti-inflammatory herbs soothes not only your back but also aching bones and muscles throughout your body.

RAW VEGETARIAN SEAFOOD: The raw vegetarian food of the sea was the first nutrition and remains of great benefit. For example, kelp, dulse, arame, hijiki and wakame have invaluable nutrients — especially minerals and trace minerals. All these foods build bone and tissue, benefiting not only your back but the rest of your skeleton and tissues.

ELECTROMAGNETIC THERAPY/FREQUENCY THERAPY: Noninvasive treatments such as diathermy, H-wave, TENS and others minimize pain and inflammation and their resultant swelling. These processes conduct electrons through affected areas and give them relief, sometimes permanently.

WHOLE-FOOD SUPPLEMENTATION: Magnesium, calcium, manganese, potassium, cadmium — all in organic form — help rebuild bones and nerves, reducing pain throughout the body.

MASSAGE: Many specialized massage techniques are effective in alleviating back injuries and problems. Consult a qualified practitioner to implement this therapy.

SAUNAS, STEAMBATH, WHIRLPOOLS: All these detoxifying treatments relax muscles, organs and other systems of the body as well as your spirit. Varying the sequence of these therapies is the best way to maximize their effects. Treat yourself to at least one of these soothing solutions at least three times a week.

ALTERNATIVE NON-SURGICAL TREATMENTS: DRX9000 is a technological remedy against back pain; this non-invasive process is a medical resource that uses NASA technology developed to regulate the fluids and ease the spines of astronauts during and after their flights. It is distributed by Axiom Worldwide, whose research indicates that cervical decompression is 86 percent as effective and can be a desirable alternative to back surgery.

BLADDER INFECTIONS

Bladder infections are becoming increasingly more commonplace because of the prevalence of E coli and other bacteria in the vagina (from which men can contract them). When these microbes enter the urinary tract, they often cause bladder infections.

PURE FLUIDS: Drink plenty of molecularly organized or distilled water, fresh green-vegetable juice, sprout juice, and some medicinal herbal teas (for example, the teas of cranberry leaf, fenugreek, and una da gato); by doing so, you will hydrate the cells of the body, stimulating and flushing the bladder and purging it of toxins.

BIO-ORGANIC CRANBERRY JUICE, CRANBERRY EXTRACTS, CRANBERRY SEEDS: The balanced acidic content of this nutritious berry stabilizes the Ph level of the contents of the bladder, creating an environment that destroys bacteria and inhibits the formation of new ones.

WHOLE-FOOD SUPPLEMENTS and HERBS: The orally ingested combination of whole food vitamin C, CoQ10 and alpha-lipoic acid enhances the immune system to combat bladder infections. These supplements can also be emulsified in water and used as a vaginal implant, to be held for three to five minutes. Sovereign silver is another powerful enemy of infections of every bodily organ. Spray three times under the tongue, and hold for two or three minutes; do so three to five times a day.

HOT GINGER BATHS: Fill your tub with warm water while you pour one-half cup of powdered ginger into it, then soak for 30 minutes. This soothing bath will alleviate stress, discomfort and pain.

REGULAR URINATION: You need not endure urinary distress, especially before and after intercourse. Regular urination cleanses the bladder, helping to eliminate infectious organisms.

GENERAL HYGIENE: The following basic elements of general hygiene benefit your health, appearance and self confidence: Wear organic cotton underwear; wear as little clothing as necessary while remaining appropriate and proper, allowing fresh air to touch your body, especially the parts of it that are usually covered.

HIGH BLOOD PRESSURE/HYPERTENSION

Hundred of millions of people throughout the world suffer from high blood pressure/hypertension. Among the causes of this serious problem are excess weight, stress, kidney dysfunction, and chronic consumption of salts, alcohol, tobacco and other addictive substances.

HAPPINESS: A study conducted at Cornell University Medical Center indicates that emotions affect blood pressure levels; the study showed that anxiety, both in people at home and outside it, increases blood pressure and hypertension and the potential for cardiovascular and other problems. Those who are relatively anxiety-free generally tend to have fewer health problems, including increased blood pressure and hypertension.

CONTEMPLATION, MEDITATION, PRAYER: Silent reflection calms the nerves and focuses your consciousness, because it secretes positive endorphins in the brain to soothe the body. Researchers at the University of Maryland discovered that when we are at rest our blood pressure is lower, but that when we communicate, orally (or even in sign language), blood pressure increases by 10 to 50 percent. So, it appears that silence is indeed golden, particularly during our golden years.

PETS and PEOPLE: Pets of all sorts, including birds and fish, give us the opportunity to be loving, responsible and positively interactive; their calming influence also reduces stress, stabilizing blood pressure and minimizing hypertension. Interaction with other people should be equally harmonious, affording everyone the peaceful existence that is best for all.

NATURE: Communing with nature nurtures your spirit, relaxes your mind, and tames your emotions. This calm manifests itself in reduced tension.

VEGAN DIET: What you eat and drink has the potential to affect you in every way possible, from complete support to absolute destruction. The obvious and logical thing to do is to sustain your best self with your best food, the banquet of exclusively vegan bio-organic delights. The implementation of this diet in conjunction with the rest of this health-promoting program not only exalts your entire body but also neutralizes any possibility of hypertension and high blood pressure. Noted physicians Dr. Neil Barnard, Dr. Dean Ornish and Dr. John McDougall have conducted extensive individual research involving blood pressure and cardiovascular disease. The results of their work indicate that the combination of a vegan diet and relaxation techniques eradicates most stress-related disorders.

HEALTHY KIDNEYS: In addition to the severe scourges of bad diet, inadequate exercise and intense stress, the most likely causes of high blood-pressure and hypertension are kidney disorders, which have three major causes:

1. Chronic dehydration, usually caused either by insufficient consumption of pure fluids or by excess consumption of alcohol.

2. Excess consumption of proteins, caused primarily either by the consumption of meat and dairy or of indigestible protein powders.

3. Pharmaceutical drugs, which deplete and damage kidney function and impair the cleansing and purification of the body. Among the many such toxic "drugs" are most steroids and most pain-killers.

EXERCISE: One of the best ways to alter hypertension is aerobic exercise done at least five days per week for 35 minutes.

NATURAL REMEDIES: Such natural substances as cayenne pepper, capsicum tincture, ginkgo biloba, garlic, cinnamon, and wheatgrass regulate blood pressure and calm the system.

BRONCHITIS AND OTHER RESPIRATORY PROBLEMS

Like colds, bronchitis is caused by a virus; therefore, antibiotics are of little use in combating it. However, many natural remedies are available for bronchitis and other respiratory problems.

AVOID ALL SMOKE: Fumes impair breathing. This means we must avoid not only the poisonous smoke from cigarettes, cigars and pipes, but that which emanates from aerosol cans, vehicles including everything from buses to airplanes, factories, commercial agriculture, and conventional trash disposal. Not only should you not smoke, but you must also avoid being around people who do.

WARM PURE FLUIDS: Drinking herbal teas such as those of eucalyptus leaf, peppermint, lemon grass, cinnamon and clove encourages the hydration and vaporization of mucus, which clears the bronchial passages. Since warm lemon water is alkalizing, it serves the same purifying function.

HUMIDIFIERS: Humid air helps release bronchial mucus; this process can be expedited by mixing tea tree oil and/or eucalyptus oil into the water in the humidifier.

HEALTHY DIET: Avoiding wheat products, dairy products, meat, and all fried or processed "food" is beneficial not only to your total health but also to relieve and prevent respiratory disorders.

PEACEFUL OUTDOOR RECREATION: Spend as much time as possible in a natural environment, deeply breathing clean air while you revel in the world around you.

RELAXATION: Avoid stress, promote harmony, and emphasize calm. Interact harmoniously with everyone and everything. Stress causes distress of bronchial function; remember how difficult it is to breathe when you become angry, frustrated or fearful.

CANCERS

Cancer is a frightening plague of contemporary times. Among the most severe of these virulent, life-destroying saboteurs are carcinomas, sarcomas, melanomas and leukemias. These mutagens have proliferated as a result of our shoddy, high-speed lives conducted in a man-made, chemically saturated, toxically polluted, ironically unlivable world. In our efforts to combat microbes we have created chemicals that cause cancer, and almost everything we eat, drink, wear and breathe can attack and destroy our health. But we can fight this scourge in various ways, as research, education and lifestyle at The Hippocrates Health Institute has proven over decades.

LIVING FOOD DIET: Uncooked vegan bio-organic food nourishes the body as it neutralizes cancers. You must emphasize the consumption of green vegetables and sprouts in order to enrich and enhance the phytochemical bank within your body that contributes to the prevention and limitation of all forms of cancer.

VIGOROUS EXERCISE: To excise toxins, you must exercise the body. In doing so, you serve a fourfold purpose: Elevating body temperature, thus destroying mutagens; eliminating waste and counterproductive cells from the body; activating endorphins that create calm and balanced metabolism; and increasing both the number and strength of the immune system's cells.

PHYSICAL THERAPIES: Hyperthermia, saunas, steam baths, Jacuzzis, oxygen therapies, and others contribute to the reduction both of the number and the effects of mutagenic cells.

PSYCHOLOGICAL THERAPIES: Psychoneuroimmunology, visualization techniques, healing affirmations and other positive psychological approaches are effective in both reducing and eliminating every kind of cancer.

COLD SORES; CHICKEN POX;
GENITAL HERPES; SHINGLES (HERPES SIMPLEX)

These viral eruptions attack individual areas of the body as well as its entirety. On the lips, they are called cold sores; their systematic lesions during childhood are known as chicken pox; on the genitalia, they constitute herpes; when they are systematic, they are called shingles and both assault the torso and travel throughout the body.

HEALTHY LIVING: A bio-organic vegan diet is the start of your self-protection against herpes simplex. Do both aerobic and resistance exercises consistently, avoid stress, keep a positive attitude, and interact harmoniously with everyone and everything. Healthy living not only makes you feel your best, but it enhances the immune system and prevents the development of retro-viruses.

NATURAL SOLUTIONS: If you are plagued by any of these problems, put camphor on affected areas. Sovereign silver (silver nitrate) is an effective topical and internal deterrent, and lysine retards the spread of these invaders. Varro E. Tyler, Ph.D., Professor of Medicine at Purdue University, suggests you rinse your mouth with potassium chlorate in water several times per day (do *not* swallow!). This procedure combats oral manifestations of herpes simplex. These and other natural solutions to viral diseases are readily available throughout the world.

HERBAL REMEDIES: You can apply goldenseal root powder directly to areas infected by herpes simplex. You can also mix it with water to use as a mouthwash which can be swallowed after use. Pau d'arco can be used as a salve on the affected area or steeped in water while left in the sun to be consumed as a non-cooked sun tea between two and five times a day.

HEALTHY DIET: Avoid any food that can compromise your immune system or intensify the effect of the herpes virus. Among such "foods" are chocolate, citrus fruits, strawberries, walnuts, coffee, and all meat — a category that includes chicken and fish.

PROBIOTICS: These healthy supplements are made of beneficial bacteria. As they circulate throughout your system, they attack herpes simplex and other microbes while enhancing the immune system so that it can continue the battle.

CELLULITE

The unsightly, undesirable, unhealthy and unnecessary problem of cellulite is caused by a combination of fat globules, waste matter, and water that is imprisoned in connective tissue. While cellulite has been associated with aging, it now ravages those of every age, including youngsters who are often under-active and mostly overweight.

MASSAGE: Legitimate forms of massage help eliminate cellulite from its toxic host. The specific technique known as cellulite massage, similar to lymphatic drainage, is an effective antidote.

HERBAL WRAPS and HERBAL BATHS: Placing herbal wraps — usually consisting of seaweed and herbs — on cellulite- affected areas reduces the severity of the condition. Warm baths with seaweed and herbs are also calming and effective against cellulite.

FAR-INFRARED THERAPY: This treatment is usually conducted in a Far-infrared sauna; placing directional Far-infrared units directly on the affected area is also therapeutic.

ELIMINATE FATS: To lose excess, unhealthy weight — much of which creates cellulite — you must eliminate fats from your diet. The fats of animal-based products (meat, dairy) are the most extreme fat-bearing culprits; however, hydrogenated vegetable oils are also culpable.

COMBAT CONSTIPATION: Constipation causes cellulite by increasing lipid levels and polluting the bloodstream. Constipation is unlikely if your diet includes enough fiber, sprouted grains, green vegetables, and green sprouts. You should also drink beverages at room temperature instead of cold, because cold beverages constrict the digestive enzymes of the esophagus and the stomach. The elimination of constipation and the incorporation of regularity are also beneficial to your general health.

CHOLESTEROL-RELATED PROBLEMS

Maintaining cholesterol balance is an essential aspect of health; so, while we need healthy cholesterol, excessive and harmful cholesterol must be excluded from our diets and bodies. The cholesterol in our food is all animal-based; a single egg contains 275 milligrams of cholesterol; an apple has none. Most responsible medical and governmental sources recommend that we consume no more than 300 milligrams of cholesterol per day. After decades of research and practical experience, I have concluded that no level of cholesterol is even remotely safe if it is derived from animal-based toxins. We require very little cholesterol; the body itself produces what it needs. Excess cholesterol causes hypertension, heart disease, strokes, phlebitis, diabetes, osteoporosis, and many other serious health problems. Contemporary scientific discoveries reveal that arterial inflammation causes as many vascular disorders as cholesterol, but the inflammation itself is caused by cholesterol as it smothers vascular tissue and precipitates infection.

LIVING-FOOD VEGAN DIET: Fresh uncooked bio-organic vegetarian foods do not burden you with dietary cholesterol. The nutritional support system inherent in this diet actually strengthens the immune system, helping combat infections and other disorders and sustaining health. The Living Food Diet is the best way to defeat any cholesterol-related problem.

EXERCISE: Expending energy doing aerobic exercise for a minimum of 35 minutes five to seven times a week strengthens heart functioning, circulation, detoxification and elimination, and elevates body temperature, causing excess cholesterol to melt. Research at The Institute has proven that the combination of aerobic exercise and a living food diet flushes cholesterol from the body eight times faster than diet without exercise.

WHOLE-FOOD SUPPLEMENTS: Research and application indicate that whole-food forms of niacin, vitamin E, vitamin C, calcium, lemongrass oil, blue-green algae and activated charcoals all help to reduce cholesterol.

SPROUTED PURIFIERS: Sprouted oats, barley, spelt, kamut, rice, and teff not only provide your body with invigorating nutrition but also help to purge it of cholesterol.

PURE LIQUIDS: Drink only molecularly organized or distilled water, fresh raw juices and herbal teas. Avoid coffee because, as research conducted by Barry R. Davis, M.D., of the University of Texas Health Science Center in Houston indicates, consumption of coffee increases cholesterol. After studying more than 9,000 people, he concluded that the volume of cholesterol increases significantly among those who drink two or more cups of coffee a day. Other studies indicate that even organic decaffeinated coffee causes similar increases. As reported in *The British Journal of Medicine*, soda pop causes not only higher levels of cholesterol but obesity and dental problems.

GARLIC: Regular consumption of significant quantities of raw garlic reduces harmful blood fats, whereas cooked garlic loses most of its cholesterol-combating potency.

COLDS and INFLUENZA

Although colds and influenza are historic plagues upon humanity, humans have found no absolute cures for them. The best we can do to combat these invaders is to live in harmony with nature and strengthen our immune systems.

INTENSIFY IMMUNITY: Proper attitude, diet and exercise constitute the foundation of health; they are critical elements of protection from influenza, common colds and all other diseases.

HOME REMEDIES: You can do a great deal at home to insulate yourself and your family from disease. For example, you can combat and even eliminate flu and colds with saunas, hot baths, footbaths, Epsom salt and ginger soaks, adequate rest and calming activities.

CONSUMPTION of PURE FLUIDS: Fresh juices made from jicama, cucumber, burdock root, garlic and ginger help remedy viral infections.

HERBAL and NUTRITIONAL SOLUTIONS: Oral applications of liquid extracts of the herb osha four to six times a day help alleviate the common cold. Drinking licorice-root sun tea is a nutritious way to neutralize viruses, calm irritated throats and relieve coughs. Sovereign silver is effective in depleting the number and strength of viruses that cause these problems. The consumption of the combination of plenty of bioactive organic zinc and whole-food vitamin C helps minimize the effect and duration of these conditions. The fatty acid monolaurin has an antiviral effect and is readily available in flaxseeds and hemp seeds.

INCLUSIONS and EXCLUSIONS: In your daily routine, include plenty of fresh air, pure water (with bio organic lemon, if possible), and lots of rest and restful sleep. But exclude from your daily routine all unwholesome so-called "food," including flour products, meat, dairy, and sweets, as well as polluted and stress-inducing environments and people and man-made fibers that inhibit the body's ability to breathe and detoxify.

CONSTIPATION, DIARRHEA AND RELATED CONDITIONS

Constipation and diarrhea are prevalent in the modern world because of unhealthy living. These gastrointestinal problems can be alleviated easily in their early stages, before they cause more severe concern.

PURE FLUIDS: Most people who suffer from these conditions are dehydrated, so their problems can be addressed simply by drinking enough pure liquids. Dehydration precipitates the imbalance of the body's electrolytes and healthy bacteria; that can lead to either uncontrolled excretion or constricted retention.

ELIMINATION of IMPURITIES: Parasites, amoebae and other counterproductive life forms can also either facilitate or restrict natural elimination. The gastrointestinal system is poisoned by heavy metals, excess cholesterol, and partially digested "food," and these excesses can intensify both constipation and diarrhea. Cleansing your system is easy; just eat properly, use natural herbal and nutritional supplementation, and avoid contamination.

NATURAL LAXATIVES and HERBAL SUPPLEMENTS: Even natural laxatives require minimal usage in order to avoid dependency upon them. Senna is a reliable purgative. Herbal supplements such as fenugreek, psyllium seed, flaxseed extract and annis-seed extract regulate intestinal activity.

ENEMAS, COLONICS, NUTRITIONAL IMPLANTS: Enemas and colonics have provided purgative relief throughout history. They should always be followed by an implant of wheatgrass and/or algae to insure the retention of electrolytes. These procedures should be undertaken only as necessary.

EXERCISE: Regular exercise benefits the bowels as much as it does the rest of the body. Abdominal exercises strengthen the muscles of the intestinal tract, fortifying them and helping to alleviate eliminatory problems involving them.

STRESS RELIEF: Just as your jaw and body constrict as a result of stress, so does your interior system; therefore, stress is a frequent cause not only of constipation and diarrhea but also of diverticulitis and Crohn's disease. Rest, relax, contemplate and interact with nature daily in order to soothe your body.

DENTAL and ORAL CONCERNS: PROBLEMS of the MOUTH AND TEETH

The human mouth contains more microbes and spirochetes than that of any other creature. That daunting reality combined with negligent personal hygiene causes severe oral and dental problems throughout life.

These problems are also involved in such disorders as heart disease, liver disease, diabetes, miscarriage, premature birth, and septic conditions (toxemia), among others.

REGULAR DENTAL CARE — DOMESTIC and PROFESSIONAL: Care of your teeth, gums and mouth is a serious daily responsibility. Even if you fulfill it well, you need to visit an experienced natural dental professional regularly. You must floss after each meal, brush with a soft medium brush using natural anti microbial compounds, and use high-pressure water projection to stimulate and cleanse gums, mouth and teeth. You should also massage your gums frequently, using hygienic methods and sanitary instruments. Your teeth must be regularly examined by a capable dentist and cleaned by an experienced dental hygienist to remove accumulated plaque.

DEPRESSION (MELANCHOLIA)

Humans have cultivated the self-sabotaging cycle of doing depressing things, thus depressing ourselves; that in turn causes us to do more depressing things, which is even more depressing. You get the picture. However, this increasingly depressing cycle can be reversed by healthy, positive living. Every form of despair — from moderate despondency to melancholia to bipolar (manic) depression — can be addressed by simple means.

HARMONIOUS RELATIONSHIPS: It is impossible to feel bad when you feel good about yourself and everyone around you, so healing your depression starts with self-esteem. Once you have achieved it, you must seek and maintain harmonious relationships with everyone and everything, including family, friends, pets, neighbors, co-workers and acquaintances.

Fulfilling relationships, whether formal or intimate, contribute profoundly to the balanced metabolism and perception that foster mental health and validated optimism.

PROFESSIONAL COUNSELING: Legitimate psychotherapy motivates the patient to focus on the positive; this procedure is of benefit in cases of depression. An expert practitioner can curb the patient's depression without traumatizing him. During the past several decades, many gifted mental-health practitioners have been valuable assets to the faculty of The Institute; and I have been fortunate enough to observe both their remarkable work and its liberating results.

GASTROINTESTINAL HEALTH: Modern research reveals that most of the body's serotonin (the internal chemistry that regulates mood and induces positive attitude) is created in the gastrointestinal tract. Keeping your intestines clean through proper diet and hydration is a significant contribution to your battle against depression.

ADEQUATE SLEEP and OTHER REST: Your brain, heart and entire body require regular rest to detoxify, reconstitute and reinvigorate. Proper sleep regulates the endorphin activity of the brain, alleviating depression. If you sleep well enough and long enough, you will be energetic and functional throughout the day, curtailing the sense of inactivity and inadequacy that mark most depressive states.

EXERCISE: All healthy physical activity — aerobic and other exercise, dancing, swimming, lovemaking, walking, and non- competitive athletics — increase positive body chemistry, often providing the balancing element that elevates one from depression. Research at Hippocrates proves that regular aerobic exercise alleviates at least half of all forms of depression.

NATURAL SUPPLEMENTATION: Phycomin algae extract beneficially affects those parts of the brain that induce depression. Extracts of kava kava extract and St. John's wort combat negativity and foster positive attitudes. And many proteins, including GABA and tryptophan, also help alleviate despair and pessimism.

EAR PROBLEMS and EYE PROBLEMS
(Infection; hearing loss; tinnitus)
(Diminishing vision; cataracts; glaucoma;
macular degeneration; infection)

Vision and hearing are two of the five glorious senses. If we are lucky enough to have them, we need to protect them so they can be a part of our longevity; the loss of either is a calamity. Modern life is often intolerably noisy, causing not only auditory distress but also diminution of hearing, ear infections and tinnitus. Often the pollutants of modern life find their way into the ear canal, causing infections that permanently impede our ability to hear.

Similarly, our eyes our bombarded by toxins and microbes, causing tearing, irritation, tissue damage, infection, temporary blindness and declining vision. Our usual ally, the sun, can be severely damaging to the eyes if they are exposed to its full power without protection. Eyes also suffer from bad digestive and eliminatory processes, which cause macular degeneration, cataracts and glaucoma. Eventually even the accumulation of pollutants and pressure in a clogged excretory system reach the eyes, causing many of vision problems.

PROPER LIVING: If you live well, you treat your senses well. The combination of a bio-organic vegan diet, positive attitude, healthy aerobic and resistance exercise and proper rest insures increased immunity and improved sensory capability.

CLEANSING THE EYES AND EARS: These delicate organs require careful daily maintenance. You must clean your eyes with such herbal solutions as cornflower at least once a day, and consumption of the herb eyebright (named for its benefits to the eyes) strengthens vision. You must do ear candling two or three times a year, and garlic oil and/or saline solutions help alleviate ear infections.

EXERCISE for EYES and EARS: The Bates Method is a series of daily eye exercises that maintain and improve vision. Hearing can be improved via exposure to harmonious natural sounds and good music, refining both the outer and inner ear and reinforcing auditory endurance.

PROTECTION: Protect your eyes with anti-glare glasses that deflect UV rays. Protect your ears from high-frequency irritation with ear plugs, and from frostbite and other cold weather hazards by covering them during inclement weather.

FATIGUE

Stress, anxiety, depression and overwork tire everyone, and the modern world drains us of our vital energy. Non-nutritive and counter-nutritive "food," sleep deprivation, depression, lethargy, environmental pollution (including noise and stench), and disorders such as Epstein-Barr virus (chronic fatigue syndrome) steal our vigor and weaken us. When we try to escape from these depleting forces, we cannot, because our rest — especially our sleep — is a source of fatigue rather than of rejuvenation.

POSITIVE ATTITUDE: Positive thought provides the confidence that motivates you to be at your best. All recovery from negativity starts with a turn toward the positive. We must realize that depression and despair are temporary enemies that fade in the light of affirmative belief and functioning.

ENERGY in MOTION: Movement is natural; lethargy is unnatural. We need to put our energy into motion at every opportunity in every positive way possible: Walk, dance, swim, glide, play, make love.

HEALTHY DIET: A rich diet of pure fluid living vegan food stimulates our glands and organs to energize us fully, while the complex carbohydrates in sprouted grains and beans nourish, fortify and energize us.

PROPER REST AND SLEEP: Depleted energy demands rest, and rest renews energy. We need both; if we lose either, we cannot function completely. Most adults require about eight hours of uninterrupted sleep nightly, so make sure you sleep neither less nor much more: Too little sleep sabotages your health and vitality; too much indicates that you are depressed and lethargic. If you sleep too little, adjust your schedule. If you sleep too much, enhance your activities.

HARMONIOUS RELATIONSHIPS: Stress between and among people deprives everyone of vigor and productivity. Eat well, exercise properly and think positively, and you will interact harmoniously whenever possible and shun disharmony whenever necessary.

FEVERS

Fevers are symptoms of infection, and lengthy or high fevers can lead to death. You are likely to have few or no fevers if you live The Longevity Program. If you or a family member has a serious fever — even a moderate one — for any length of time, see a caring, competent medical practitioner.

HEALTHY LIQUIDS: Drink plenty of either distilled or molecularly organized water with the juice of one bio-organic lemon per liter (1 quart). Drink 12 ounces (360 milliliters) of fresh raw green juices at least three times daily, and avoid dairy, coffee, alcohol, soda pop, fruit juices, carrot juice, beet juice and everything containing sugar.

COMPRESSES and SPONGE BATHS: Take a towel made of natural fibers, soak it in ice-cold water, and apply it to the forehead for 15 minutes. Alternate with a hot compress every 15 minutes, continuing the sequence until the fever drops. If the fever reaches or exceeds 37 degrees Celsius (103 degrees Fahrenheit), exclude the hot compress but continue the cold. Take a sponge made of natural fibers, soak it in ice-cold water, pat the forehead and other feverish areas for at least 20 minutes and continue as long as necessary to bring relief. The resulting evaporation cools the body and lowers its temperature.

BATHS: Put 10 drops each of the following essential oils into a hot bath: Spearmint, tea tree and eucalyptus. Soak for 30 minutes while applying a cold compress to the forehead. This soothing process helps diminish fevers. Note: If the fever reaches or exceeds 37 degrees Celsius (103 degrees Fahrenheit), do not bathe in hot water. A tubful of warm water with 15 drops of pure rosewater in it also help relieve fevers associated with colds and flu, as can very warm sea-salt footbaths in a container that accommodates both feet, in which very warm water. Put 15 drops of pure rosewater into a tubful of warm water. Footbaths are also useful against fevers. Pour very warm water into a container that can accommodate both feet and soak them for 15 to 30 minutes.

WARM VAPOR: Both traditional and modern means of vaporization fight not only fevers but also colds, flu and other respiratory problems. In the traditional approach, place a towel over the head; then carefully lean over a teapot of boiling water, allowing its vapor to permeate the nostrils for 10 to 20 minutes. Modern vaporizers can be placed in the room where the affected persons sleeps, allowing it to work through the night. You may add favorite essential oils to either process.

RAW VEGAN FOOD: The following vegetables (among others) have significant water content: Cucumbers, winter squash, celery, rutabaga and jicama. Their water content helps alleviate fevers by nourishing weakened cells.

FOOT PROBLEMS

Like the rest of the body, the feet are important to health and functioning. Unfortunately, they are often disregarded, mistreated and even abused, as in the ancient and brutal practice of foot-binding, which ruins women's feet for life as well as compromising their circulation, mobility, appearance and self-respect. As a result, both the bound feet and the victim's self-regard often degenerate with age. Among the many other plagues to which our feet are subjected are fungal and bacterial infections, corns, hammertoes, arch disorders, constricted circulation (pedal neuropathy), and ingrown toenails.

PROPER FOOT CARE: Hygiene must be universal; you must apply it lovingly to your entire body. When you bathe or shower, lather your feet with natural soap; then, spend at least two or three minutes rubbing your feet vigorously with a brush that has natural bristles. Clip nails (of both feet and hands) regularly and carefully. Be careful: If you cut the corners of your toenails too closely, you will cause ingrown toenails, while cutting too closely across your nails will cause irritation, infection and discomfort. Maintain and invigorate your cuticles regularly. Frequent foot massage is both pleasant and healthy. When done professionally, it is called reflexology, but you can massage your own feet. If you are fortunate enough to be in a loving relationship, affectionate massage is one of its rewards. If you like, you can intensify the experience by applying bio-organic lotions and creams to soften skin, thereby combating and preventing calluses.

PROPER FOOTWEAR: Many of us clothe our bodies with care but cover our feet carelessly. The result is a lifetime of discomfort, distortion, contortion, pain, and unnecessarily unsightly feet. Many shoes constrain the feet, causing unnatural development and various infections. Like the rest of the body, the feet must breathe, but most footgear does not allow much breathing at all. Imagine, say, an eight-hour workday with an hour of travel each way. For your feet, that means at least ten hours without air.

Stilettos are among the most barbaric footwear. Like all high-heeled shoes, they cause not only foot pain but also severe discomfort in the calves, thighs and back. Solely for appearance, many women endure profound agony.

Ballet shoes may look attractive and comfortable, but they do not offer enough support to feet or ankles. In addition, ballet itself is an unnatural activity foisted upon children as young as five. Eventually the practice permanently distorts the foot — especially the toes — as well as causing problems to the legs and lower back.

If you wear shoes, wear shoes that allow your feet to breathe, your blood to circulate and your movements to be free. The shoes that allow your feet to breathe most completely are sandals, but do not wear shoes any longer than necessary, and when appropriate wear clean socks made of natural materials. Best of all, walk barefoot whenever possible.

PROPER ACTIVITIES: As we said, ballet is destructive to feet. Similarly, competitive gymnastics requiring participants to fly through the air before landing often cause broken ankles, feet, and toes. If you are going to ski or skate, make sure that your footgear is appropriate for both your feet and the activity. If you plan to dance for any length of time, wear comfortable shoes; women should not wear high heels for dancing.

ENSURE PROPER CIRCULATION: Since blood must travel further to your hands and feet than to any other part of your body, you must ensure its proper circulation by, among other things, a healthy aerobic exercise program, swimming, sunbathing, proper nutrition, adequate rest and the use of stimulating herbal creams and essential oils and massage.

HERPES

Genital herpes has become a worldwide epidemic. Other forms of herpes such as chicken pox, cold sores, and shingles are also prevalent. Each of these viral infections has potentially severe effects.

SAFE SEX: Romance is a fundamental physical and emotional component of mature life. However, we must be self- protective before we undertake it. You must respect yourself sufficiently to interact only with those who themselves have enough self-respect to protect you. This means an open and honest exchange of personal information before intimacy is initiated. If you cannot have complete trust in your potential sexual partner, you must serve your permanent health before your temporary pleasure.

SUPPLEMENTS: Organic bioactive lysine, either taken internally or applied externally, helps prevent the outbreak of herpes. Camphor applied topically helps reduce the duration and intensity of herpetic infection.

AVOID EXTREME CLIMACTIC CONDITIONS: Extremes of weather — too sunny or too cold — weaken the immune system, allowing the spread of the herpes virus throughout your system.

AVOID ACID-FORMING FOODS: Too much acid in your system gives the herpes virus an open field for infestation. Many foods infest your system by forming excess acid in it; among these foods are unripe citrus, tomatoes, pineapples, rhubarb, and jalapeno peppers.

IMPECCABLE IMMUNITY: When you strengthen your immune system with healthy living, a refined raw diet, proper exercise and positive attitude, you combat not only herpes but also all other plagues that oppress us.

HEADACHES

Almost half of us worldwide suffer from headaches of various types. Most are caused by digestive disorders, stress, pollution including noise, allergies, eyestrain (often caused by extensive focus on television screens, computer monitors and video games), and improper or insufficient sleep.

PROPER SLEEP: As we have discussed, sleep is critical to health. Sleep has three purposes: to rest, detoxify and reconstitute the body; to rest and reinvigorate the mind by restructuring the brain cells into proper balance; and to facilitate cellular reconstruction of every part of the anatomy. Since these functions occur in unison, violation of any of them causes headaches and other neuronal impairments.

INTESTINAL CLEANSING: Many headaches are caused by dysfunctions of digestion and elimination. Each of these discomforts causes extreme acidity, which pollutes the bloodstream, reducing the supply of oxygen to the brain.

AVOID ALL POLLUTION, INCLUDING NOISE: Inhalation and absorption of the many chemical pollutants in our environment causes intense headaches and severe eye pain. These toxins are emitted by gasoline, hairsprays, perfumes and colognes, cleaning products, chlorine bleach and many other environmental contaminants. Pollution violates not only our sense of sight but also — in our time, especially — our sense of hearing. Our ears suffer permanent damage from the constant noises of traffic (including trains and airplanes), incessant construction, shrill audio systems, loud individuals and groups, and all of the other oppressive and unsound sound-blasts to which we are subjected daily. These auditory irritations not only cause headaches but increase blood pressure and stress and interfere with our rest.

AVOID "FOOD" ADDITIVES: Much of our modern "food" is fouled by chemical preservatives and taste enhancers; among the worst of these are dyes and other artificial forms of coloring, sugar substitutes such as aspertame, salt substitutes such as MSG, stabilizers and fortifiers, oxygen depleting fats and other.

EXERCISE: Proper aerobic exercise, especially when done in natural surroundings, helps reduce stress and fill the brain with oxygen, thus preventing and alleviating headaches.

HARMONIOUS INTERACTION: How often have you heard or said such phrases as, "My work gives me a headache" or "My life is one big headache"? Unfortunately, like most clichés, the phrases are all too often true. But since peace starts within each of us, we can cure not only headaches but many other personal, familial, professional, social and environmental problems by interacting harmoniously with all of life.

HEARTBURN, ACID REFLUX AND OTHER ACIDIC CONDITIONS

While pollution attacks us from the outside, excess acidity literally eats away at our insides. The stomach often forces its acids into the esophagus, causing acid reflux disease. Usually, this process is a component of an excessively acidic system. Excess acidity also promotes and intensifies disease (including esophagal cancer) and generates intense pain for long periods.

HEALTHY DIET: To reduce the impact of excess acidity, you must live The Longevity Diet, eliminate acid forming liquids from your menu (for example, coffee, tea, soda pop), and consume raw apple cider vinegar.

HERBAL SOLUTIONS and MINERAL SOLUTIONS: Take prescribed focal herbal medications and/or minerals as long as necessary. Among the best herbal remedies are ginger root, bitters, fenugreek, aloe vera, and flaxseed water. Among the best mineral remedies are ionic liquid forms of calcium, magnesium and potassium. (Use calcium carbonate, if possible.)

DETOXIFYING THERAPIES: Saunas, steam baths, whirlpools and other soothing treatments calm not only your exterior but also the acidity in your system. If you are new to these therapies, use each of them for three to five minutes at least once a day, five to sever days a week; as you use them regularly, you can increase the time to as much as 15 minutes. Drink plenty of pure water both during and after these calming sessions.

NEUROMUSCULAR MASSAGE: This form of bodywork specifically invigorates muscles and other tissues, purging the cells and glands of excess acid content.

INSOMNIA

Lack of sleep, improper sleep, and interrupted sleep are among the most severe problems of our time. Violated sleep interferes with health, schedules, productivity, patience, and joy. As we age, many of us have increasingly severe problems falling asleep. Throughout this book (especially in this chapter) you will read discussions of proper sleep as a solution to all sorts of problems, so we need not reiterate them here except to emphasize again and again that healthy, appropriate, sufficient sleep is essential to everything that we do.

IRRITABLE BOWEL SYNDROME AND OTHER INTESTINAL DISORDERS

Stress and improper diet cause more problems today than ever; among them are such intestinal irritations as diarrhea, constipation and abdominal pain, individually or in combinations. These problems are intensified by reckless high-speed living.

PROPER DIET: You must eliminate all meats, dairy and flour products, alcohol and caffeinated beverages from your diet. In your healthy new diet, include fresh green juices, fresh raw green vegetables, flaxseed, psyllium seed, fenugreek sprouts and cabbage sprouts.

SUPPLEMENTS: Raw aloe vera juice, used orally or rectally, relaxes the bowels. Iberogast, a well-known European herbal combination, is an effective remedy for bowel irritations. Take a half-dropper of liquid fenugreek extract three to five times a day as needed.

REDUCED STRESS: Avoid conflict, distress, anxiety, inharmonious environments, and anything else that sabotages your sense of peace. Interact in harmony with nature and all of life; contemplate, meditate, pray; rest appropriately and well; make positive, life-affirming decisions and take positive, life-affirming actions.

SPEED-WALKING AND OTHER EXERCISE: The invigorating exercise known as speed-walking activates endorphins, reducing stress, irritation and pain. Regular healthy exercise calms the bowels and improves their functioning.

INTERNAL AND EXTERNAL APPLICATION OF FLUIDS: Always drink adequate amounts of pure liquids — distilled and/or molecularly organized water and the juices of raw vegetables and sprouts. When necessary, take a pure-water enema followed immediately by four ounces (120 milliliters) of either freshly prepared wheatgrass juice or frozen and thawed blue-green algae and retain it for approximately 15 20 minutes. This application re-mineralizes your gastrointestinal tract and supports your electrolytes instead of draining them. It also provides oxygen-rich chlorophyll to help heal the intestines.

KIDNEY STONES; GALL STONES LIVER STONES; BLADDER STONES

Stones lodged in a vital organ are among the most painful afflictions of the human body. They are, of course, not actually stones, but accumulations of calcified undigested lipids and minerals. Most such stones can be excised naturally; however, some of them must be medically addressed, either through non-invasive lithotripsy or, as a last resort, surgery. Before you resort to any extreme measure, try the following natural solutions:

BIO-ORGANIC CRANBERRY JUICE OR CRANBERRY-JUICE EXTRACT: Consume fresh raw bio-organic cranberry juice or cranberry juice extract to combat kidney stones and bladder stones. The acidity in cranberries helps to erode the "stones" in these water-based organs.

FLUSHING of the LIVER and GALLBLADDER: Useful if your organs are healthy and you do not have hepatitis, liver cancer, gallbladder cancer or cirrhosis. Before flushing, fast for three days by drinking raw green juices and small amounts of the juice of bio-organic apples thoroughly diluted in pure water. On the third night of your fast, before you go to sleep, drink one-half cup of pure hemp oil, flax oil or olive oil, mixed with the juice of two bio-organic lemons and four to six cloves of compressed garlic. When you awaken, drink 1 liter (1 quart) of lemon water or diluted bio-organic apple juice (it should be 10 parts distilled water to one part apple juice). Your body will prompt you to clear the bowels; do so. You should find eliminated "stones" in the toilet bowl. PLEASE NOTE: This procedure requires the involvement of a compassionate, knowledgeable practitioner.

HEALTHY EATING: Keeping all your organs healthy and unclogged means living The Longevity Diet: You must not consume animal-based products, cooked oils, or any fried or processed "foods."

PROPER EXERCISE: Stretching, aerobics and resistance exercise all help purge the body of the excess accumulated debris that becomes these "stones."

ACUPUNCTURE and SHIATSU MASSAGE: Acupuncture stimulates the meridian (the electrical circuitry of the body), creating the peristaltic purging that helps eliminate these toxic clusters. Shiatsu massage helps to stretch the ligaments and muscles, forcing excess toxic debris out of the body.

FAR-INFRARED HEAT: Directional Far-infrared heat (produced by placing a therapeutic apparatus on the affected organ) generates thermal healing throughout the body to soften the stones and make them easier to discharge. Use Far-infrared heat before any other approach whenever possible. (Although Far-infrared saunas are more readily available than directional far-infrared heat, they are not as stimulating.)

MENOPAUSAL DISTRESS

Historically, menopause initiated at maturity; for many women today, it begins at much younger ages. PMS (premenstrual syndrome) also oppresses more than half our female population during their years of menstruation. Internationally, the respected anthropologist Margaret Mead said that mature women benefit from PMZ — Post-Menopausal Zest. Dr. Mead encouraged women to greet their mature years with enthusiasm, vigor and joy, and she emphasized constructive post-menstrual developments such as the end of the monthly cycle, the lack of fear of pregnancy and the accompanying freedom from contraceptive devices. She concluded that this stage of life provides a woman with enormous freedom.

CLOTHES MADE OF NATURAL FIBERS: Wearing such clothing prevents seepage of the hormone-altering environmental estrogens in manmade fibers into the body; these chemicals alter a woman's natural processes. Organic cotton, linen and hemp are your best clothing choices during menopause because they keep you cool and comfortable.

HEALTHY EXERCISE: Such invigorating activities as dancing, jumping rope, bicycling, walking and swimming balance hormones and reduce symptoms of menopause as well as increase vitality, energy, self-confidence and joy.

PROPER DIET: Eat small meals of raw bio-organic food. Drink pure liquids. And avoid all "food" that disturbs body, mind and emotions.

RETAIN ROMANTIC VITALITY: Norma McCoy, Ph.D., Professor of Psychology at San Francisco State University, has reported that women who remain sexually active during menopause have few or no "hot flashes" compared to those who have little or no romantic activity during that time. Julian M. Davis, Ph.D., Professor of Psychology at Stanford University, studied women whose menopause was beginning; he concluded that frequent romance helps to boost declining estrogen levels, thereby minimizing both the occurrence and effect of hot flashes.

MENSTRUAL CRAMPS

Just as menopausal problems are now plaguing women at younger ages, menstruation often begins during the pre-teens. This is a significant departure from historic maturation. In previous centuries, menstruation usually began during the late teens; just decades ago, it was seen in the mid-teens; and, now it is literally stealing childhoods and further complicating the already complicated early teen years. PMS was nonexistent as recently as the mid-20th century. Chemically laden foods and polluted environments are the prime culprits causing the intensified pain and distress of PMS.

POSITIVE VISUALIZATION: Women have struggled to establish positive self-image in most societies; this imposed negativity causes not only mental and emotional distress but also a biochemical lack of balance in the body that can cause premature menstruation. All of us require positive self-image as a foundation of positive functioning. Every woman needs to be able to fully respect herself so she can assume her rightful place in the social structure, as well as assure herself of proper physical development and change. See yourself at your best, and you will present yourself at your best.

WHOLE FOODS AND WHOLE-FOOD SUPPLEMENTS: A critical aspect of self-respect is a diet that respects your integrity. You need sufficient amounts of vitamins, minerals, trace minerals and proteins in your daily raw vegan diet. To ensure that your diet is complete, you can incorporate whole-food supplements into it. Choose supplements that are geared for women; they should include vitamins A, C, D, E and K, B-complex vitamins, calcium, magnesium, potassium, phosphorous, manganese, copper, zinc, algae-based proteins, and pollen-based proteins.

UNDERGARMENTS OF NATURAL FIBERS: Your underwear should be made of organic cotton or hemp, both of which facilitate ventilation and provide toxin-free comfort.

PROPER PERSONAL HYGIENE: Tending to your body hygienically serves it in many ways; among them is the cleansing and purifying of those parts of the female body that are affected by developmental changes. Too many women have become accustomed to using chemically laden, unhealthy, unsafe products for their personal hygienic needs, but not only do these products fail to sufficiently serve their supposed functions, but many also cause dysplasia (development of pre-cancerous cells), cysts, fibroid tumors, and cancer itself. Use only natural organic-cotton vaginal applications. When possible, sunbathe nude. Luxuriate in baths to which you have added such essential oils as ylang ylang, lavender, wintergreen and chamomile.

MUSCLES: PAIN, BRUISING and DEGENERATION

Our muscles make us not only strong but also secure. They assist the functioning of all bodily systems, and they ensure the integrity of our anatomy. When muscles weaken, we become emaciated, lethargic, minimally functional and unattractive. Weakened muscle structure also induces weight gain, intense pain, and disorders of digestion and elimination.

RESISTANCE EXERCISE: 82 percent of the muscles in our body feed from fat, so regular resistance exercise is imperative to attain and maintain a fit, trim, active body. When a body is too thin, the only healthy weight to be added is muscle, and this positive gain must be achieved by consistent constructive and healthy weight-lifting. Everyone of any age is capable of doing such lifting. In addition to lifting barbells, you can use weight-resistant machines, aqua-strengthening equipment, hatha yoga, callinetics, and non-competitive gymnastics. Studies at the Karolinska Institute in Stockholm prove that sports massage also assists development of muscle mass.

BODY-BUILDING DIET: It is wrongly believed that animal based "foods" and most commercial protein powders build muscle without harming the body. Both these notions are wrong —and dangerous. The best foods to build your body naturally are sprouted nuts, seeds, grains and beans, because their pre-digested amino acids course through your body quickly while heavy and indigestible "proteins" rob your body of vital energy, tax your kidneys, build no muscles and inhibit your longevity. Supplemental forms of algae and pollens also benefit your musculature without compromising your system.

THERMAL THERAPY: Whirlpools, herbal wraps, dry saunas, steam baths, and the application of tiger balm and other essential oils and lotions provide needed heat to strained or injured muscles. These therapies facilitate blood flow to damaged areas, reinvigorating and healing them.

MASSAGE: Almost all forms of massage, from Swedish to neuromuscular, benefit the muscular structure and maximize its functioning. The kneading of sore muscles expedites their healing and elongates their mass.

NAUSEA

Stress, respiratory distress caused by both internal and external toxins, various illnesses, and junk food are the primary causes of nausea. Because this is the case, each major cause can be neutralized to eliminate nausea.

REDUCE STRESS: If you live properly using The Longevity Program, your stress is reduced, as is the stress of those who come into significant contact with you. A calm system is not disturbed intestinally or in any other way. Devote significant time every day to contemplation and reflection, staying in harmony with all of life.

HERBAL SUPPLEMENTS: Disturbed intestines can be calmed with raw and powdered ginger, peppermint tea, aloe vera leaf, camomile extract and raspberry-leaf tea.

HEALTHY DIET: Consume only raw bio-organic foods; they nourish the body rather than deplete it, and they do not clog it with the toxic debris that often causes nausea.

AVOID DISTURBING SENSORY INPUT: Whenever possible, protect yourself by protecting your senses.

1. Sight: Disturbing visual images engender many negative bodily responses, including nausea.

2. Smell: Malodorous impositions provoke regurgitation and other physical distress.

3. Hearing: Sharp, irritating noise not only harms your ears permanently but can also cause vomiting.

4. Taste: The violation of our taste buds is sure to cause vomiting and other gastrointestinal distress.

5. Touch: Touching shocking or irritating objects can cause nausea.

OSTEOPOROSIS
AND OTHER SKELETAL CONCERNS

Osteoporosis (found primarily among women) is often associated with unhealthy aging; however, it need not be part of any maturing process. This disorder is caused by the modern industrialized sedentary lifestyle and is becoming more and more prevalent. Ironically, until our time skeletal degeneration was not part of aging. Today, however, many of us must endure not only osteoporosis but also bone spurs (also common among younger people), joint pain, fractures (especially from falls caused by weakened hard tissue), curvature of the spine including distorted posture, bone contortion and weakened anatomy.

RESISTANCE EXERCISE: The most effective way to combat bone degeneration and maintain strength is to do healthy and proper resistance exercise regularly. All osteoporotic conditions are caused by lack of appropriate weight-bearing activity. Not so many years ago, weight-bearing exertion was a part of every person's life; today, we are weaker because less physical lator is required of us.

BODY-STRENGTHENING FOOD: Magnesium, calcium, manganese, silica, potassium, vitamin B-12, vitamins A and D are all necessary for healthy bone development and skeletal maintenance. These and other nutrients can easily be found in a great variety of raw vegan foods, including sea-water algae, fresh-water algae, sprouted grains and grasses, leafy green vegetables and many non-sugary root vegetables such as jicama, parsnip and celeric.

WHOLE-FOOD SUPPLEMENTS: In addition to these foods, you might need such natural supplements as bioavailable silica, sea kelp tablets, whole-food calcium and magnesium, and bioactive vitamins C, A, D and B-12.

STRUCTURAL REALIGNMENT: The expert application of this form of bodywork repositions bones into their original structural patterns, facilitating the proper blood flow that assists the strengthening and maintenance of the anatomy.

PARKINSON'S DISEASE AND OTHER AUTO-IMMUNE DISEASE

Other serious health problems caused by modern living are diseases that attack the auto-immune system. Among them, and affecting everyone of any age, are multiple sclerosis (MS) and lupus.

Parkinson's disease is a chronic neurological disorder; its symptoms are systemic rigidity that causes muscular weakness, tremors, and uncontrolled movement of various parts of the body.

NEUROMUSCULAR MASSAGE: This restructuring form of bodywork is not only relaxing but also stimulates neurological function, preventing both the symptoms and the development of Parkinson's disease.

CONSUMPTION OF HEALTH-PROMOTING LIQUIDS: Raw juices made from dandelion greens, purslane, fenugreek sprouts, fennel and nasturtium flowers energize the nerves and combat the rapid degeneration that often characterizes Parkinson's. Pure water, green tea and other natural herbal drinks facilitate your body's resistance against the nerve-damaging assaults of destructive auto-immune afflictions.

WHOLE-FOOD SUPPLEMENTS: B complex vitamins, vitamin C, and the amino acid known as glutamic acid are direct antagonists of the cause and spread of Parkinson's.

ENERGIZING MOVEMENT: At every age, we need freedom of movement to maintain the energy and suppleness of body and mind. Unfortunately, upon reaching maturity some of us delude ourselves that we have earned the right to be stationary. This is foolhardy and dangerous; we need to move energetically and enthusiastically every day. Not only are walking and swimming of great value, but the pleasant resistance of walking in clean water, whether a pool or at a natural site, is exhilarating and healthy.

POSITIVE ATTITUDE: Despair and melancholia are chronic aspects of many lives. One of the most serious problems many face at maturity — often caused, ironically, by the "successful" life that allows us to retire — is the cultivation of a health-impairing hopelessness. We need instead to maintain a positive attitude, not just for our own sake but for those who care about us, and rely upon the lessons we have culled from experience.

PHLEBITIS AND OTHER VENTRICULAR PROBLEMS

Inflammation of the veins is usually caused by inactivity, high-fat diets and blood-sugar disorders. These enemies of health and function can be easily defeated, but if you have phlebitis you are at great risk for heart problems.

AEROBIC EXERCISE: Energetic movement promotes efficient blood-flow, so moderate but consistent aerobic exercise is necessary to combat phlebitis as well as other potential physical problems.

NATURAL SUPPLEMENTS: Whole-food vitamin E, chlorella (freshwater algae), supplemental pollens, whole-food niacin and potassium aid proper circulation, preventing and combating phlebitis.

VEGAN FOOD: A diet that excludes all animal-based "foods" is the only one that supports complete health; in the case of prevention and control of phlebitis, this diet is essential.

HERBAL EXTRACTS: Capsicum tincture (cayenne), ginkgo biloba, and eucalyptus oil aid circulation and help combat the unnatural coagulants that cause phlebitis.

PROSTATE PROBLEMS

Not only do prostate problems develop at every age, they are among the most epidemic concerns of modern males. These maladies include cancer, bleeding, frequent urination, pain and erectile dysfunction. Obviously, they impede the functioning and fulfillment of everyone at every age and, just as obviously, they need not continue to plague us.

HEALTHY INTIMACY: Love knows no restriction; romance knows no age. So for the health of body, mind, emotions and spirit, romance remains a delightfully life-affirming celebration. Scientific research indicates that lovemaking at least four times a week is optimal not only for prostate health but also for the partners' relationship and longevity.

HEALTHY AND HEALING DIET: A diet that includes plenty of arugula, asparagus, artichokes, cabbage sprouts, mung-bean sprouts and pumpkin-seed sprouts benefits proper functioning of the prostate. You should also drink plenty of natural green juices, pure water, and organic herbal teas. NOTE: Do not drink anything for three hours before going to sleep.

SUPPORTIVE SUPPLEMENTS: Whole-food B complex vitamins, vitamin A, phosphorous, zinc and calcium promote the functioning of the prostate as well as the other glands.

GENITAL CLIMATE CONTROL: It is important to keep the genitals warm in order to ensure proper circulation and normal urination. This supportive function requires undergarments made of natural or organic fibers. Undergarments consisting of manmade fibers are restrictive, unhealthy and irritating.

SUPPLEMENTAL ESSENTIAL FATTY ACIDS: Sunflower seeds, flaxseeds, hemp seeds, and sprouted pumpkin seeds — and their extracts — are tasty building blocks of health and maintain the prostate.

HEALING HERBS: Pygeum Africanum and saw-palmetto extracts are the most effective natural remedies for combating prostate problems.

PSORIASIS AND OTHER DERMAL IRRITATIONS

Since our skin breathes, it must be provided with oxygen and other nutrients. When it is not, various irritations occur causing us not only distress and pain but also affecting our appearance. Although most conventional practitioners claim that the causes of these maladies are unknown, they are, in fact, caused by the systemic spread of yeast and fungi.

HEALTHY/NATURAL DIET: To keep your skin and your entire system healthy, you must avoid all sugars including fruits, all flour products, cooked white potatoes, all dairy and all meats. Instead, energize your menu with germinated greens and germinated beans and all the delicious meals that we can make with them. Other healthy selections include varieties of nutritious vegetables, especially greens.

BODY THERAPIES: Epsom salt baths, dry brushing, saunas (both heat-based and Far-infrared-based), and full spectrum UV lamp therapy help reduce the problems and symptoms of psoriasis and other skin-related ailments.

SUNSHINE AND SALT-WATER BATHING: If your schedule and environment allow, enjoy the sunshine before 9 A.M. and after 4 P.M. The sodium in major bodies of water is therapeutic, as are the vitamin D-creating UV rays of the sun.

RADIATION POISONING

We have mined uranium from the beginnings of the Industrial Revolution during the mid-19th century, dispersing the vile plague of radioactivity. Radiation poisoning has insinuated itself into our air, water, food and clothing. Although we are irradiated everywhere by everything, we can do much to prevent or at least minimize the catastrophic effects of radiation.

DRINK PURE WATER: The purest water today is either distilled or molecularly organized. This H2O not only refreshes you but it hydrates radio-activated cells, helping to relieve them of that radioactivity.

GREEN FOOD: All foods that contain concentrated chlorophyll — green vegetables, most sprouts, all salt-water and fresh-water algae — have individual radioactive frequencies that help extract counterproductive radioactivity from the body.

NATURAL THERAPIES: Far-infrared saunas, clay and seaweed body-wraps, whirlpool tubs, and seaweed/ginger baths counteract the effects of radiation and heal the body after those effects.

BATHING IN SALT WATER: Bathing in natural salt water neutralizes radioactivity because the minerals in salt water draw radioactive material from the cells of the body.

RESPIRATORY DISORDERS, including such breathing problems as ALLERGIES, EMPHYSEMA, TUBERCULOSIS

Although our lungs regenerate completely every 70 days, they consist of thin, fragile, delicate tissue that requires constant hydration. If this necessity is absent (although other causes, such as viruses, bacteria, yeast, molds, tobacco, and other pollutants, might engender similar distress), our lungs can suffer scarring, collapse, severely restricted functioning, and, potentially, death.

BREATHING EXERCISES AND OTHER RELAXATION TECHNIQUES: We can do breathing exercises at every age to promote and maintain healthy lungs. We can also enjoy music, glorious environments, visual arts and enriching literature to calm the lungs as well as the rest of the system. Positive visualization techniques, meditation/contemplation/prayer, and adequate rest and sleep also contribute to proper breathing and overall functioning.

HARMONIOUS INTERACTION: Breathing is impeded by such negative behaviors as violence, frustration, confrontation, anger and other types of distress. To keep your breathing and behavior at their best, be civil, courteous, polite and happily proper.

HEALTHY DIET: Allergies to gluten and dairy products are the prevalent causes of respiratory ailments. Any "food" that creates acid throughout the body weakens respiratory function; among the worst of these are meats, unripe fruits and bakery items. For best breathing, your diet should include selections from the bio-organic banquet.

NUTRIENTS AND HERBS: To maintain and even increase the health and capacity of your lungs, consume lipase enzymes, trace minerals, silver, gold, copper, and zinc, as well as pure spearmint, eucalyptus and wintergreen oils.

SEXUAL DYSFUNCTION

Sexual incapacity is a serious concern at every age. Because romantic love is a profound need at every age, this situation must be addressed. Sexual dysfunction is most often caused by hormonal imbalance rather than emotional restriction or permanent physical incapacity. The hormonal imbalances are caused by the pollution in our chemically laden environment — air, water, "food," clothing, cosmetics. Radioactivity emitted from our watches, cell phones, portable radios, computers, and airplanes— also pollutes both our bodies and activities.

ORGANIC VEGETARIAN FOODS: If you eat well, you function well: Serve the body and it will serve you. Some natural foods have been proven to have aphrodisiacal potency; among them are lettuce, arame seaweed, hijiki seaweed, fenugreek sprouts, sesame-seed sprouts and chickpea sprouts. If you eat pure foods, you allow complete natural circulation of oxygen throughout your system, thereby permitting the full metabolic activity that enhances all physical functioning, including romance.

OTHER EXERCISE: Lovemaking is delightful in many ways, including as a vigorous exercise; to reinvigorate and promote your exercise of romance, you can do such additional athletic activities as leg-strengthening, weight-lifting, abdominal enhancement, cross-training and other exercises that promote circulation in the lower extremities.

SUPPLEMENTS FOR INTIMACY: Many natural supplements assist warmth, affection and romance; among them are whole- food B-complex vitamins, whole-food vitamin E, whole-food complete essential amino acids from such sources as pollens and algae, manganese, phosphorous and selenium.

SEXUALLY TRANSMITTED DISEASES

As we have mentioned, the immediate impetus for intimacy must be tempered by thought, understanding, candor and trust. Short-term satisfaction exchanged for long-term distress is no satisfaction at all. Know and trust your partner before you engage in intimacy. In our time, there are simply more types of sexually transmitted diseases. Some, such as gonorrhea, syphilis, HIV/AIDS, chlamydia, herpes and crabs, are well known. Others are equally virulent but less notorious; these include chronic fatigue syndrome, hepatitis, parasites and amoebae, infectious spirochetes, trichomonas and many other physical, psychological, emotional and relational diseases.

ADEQUATE PROTECTION: You must protect yourself and others not only physically but emotionally. We are all familiar with the obvious and necessary physical precautions before and during intimacy, but we must also be sensitive to those emotional cautions that prevent anger, frustration, rejection, despair and severe anxiety. As we have said, you must have complete knowledge and trust in your partner's history and veracity. If you are sure of neither but are nevertheless sure of your intense interest in another person, at least protect yourselves with the best means possible.

HEALTHY LIFESTYLE: Do everything you can to support and enhance your immune system and general functioning, including a bio-organic diet, positive attitude, healthful exercise, avoidance of addictive behavior and rational choices of partners, places and activities.

SLEEP DISORDERS

Although insufficient, disrupted and stressful sleep plagues many of us, these problems seem to be even more prevalent among those who age unhealthily. Not only do sleep problems inhibit efficiency, functioning and longevity itself, but sleep deprivation is often a cause of death. Each hour of lost sleep is one hour of lost life, according to sleep medicine pioneer William C. Dement.

PSYCHOTHERAPY: Non-traditional forms of therapy such as psychoneuroimmunology allow you to confront and neutralize long-term personal problems that cause restlessness, sleeplessness and bad dreams. Legitimate hypnosis conducted by an experienced practitioner helps you deal with issues that cause concern and stress.

HEALTHY DIET: A diet rich in minerals strengthens the nervous system and promotes neuron activity in the brain. Foods such as sea vegetables, root vegetables and raw organic seeds contribute minerals and trace minerals to the biochemical health of your system. Avoid sugars and such "foods" as bread, cakes and pasta, because they increase the sugar content of your blood to excessive levels that disturb the brain and impede all rest, especially sleep.

SUPPORTIVE SUPPLEMENTS: Blue-green algae, green algae, dulse in powder or tablet form, GABA protein and gingko biloba provide nutrients that maximize mental function and support the physical health of the brain. Among the many natural herbal supplements that aid sleep and other forms of rest are St. John's Wort, slippery elm, jin bu huan and valerian root.

EXERCISES FOR BOTH BODY AND BRAIN: Rebounding on a trampoline for 35 minutes 5 to 7 times each week activates the endorphins in the brain, harmonizes hormones, and increases the number of immune cells that the body produces, all of which contribute to restful sleep as well as to physical health. Lifting free weights also strengthens those parts of the brain that harbor depression, a leading enemy of rest and one of the major causes of sleep deprivation.

TENDONITIS

Tendon-related inflammations often become chronic. Excessive abuse of body parts, sports injuries and accidents are the three major causes of tendinitis. If it is to be ameliorated, rest must be the primary means of improvement. Many people suffer from the tendinitis of the shoulders, neck and head caused by the extreme auditory stress common in our noisy world; distressingly, these auditory assaults eventually impair our ability to hear.

ADEQUATE REST: Proper rest allows your body to relax, reducing inflammation of every part of the anatomy.

ALKALINE FOODS: Most raw living bio-organic foods have little or no acidity; they alkalize the body, reducing pain and inflammation. Raw green juices, green salads, ripe bio-organic fruits and sprouted legumes expedite the process that heals you of tendinitis.

BODY THERAPIES: Deep muscle massage, Rolfing, structural alignment, shiatsu and other such therapies relax, reinvigorate and normalize the tendons. Acupuncture and acupressure help to diffuse the unpleasant tenderness caused by this disorder.

WATER EXERCISE: Relaxed swimming in warm water neutralizes the gravitational pressures that aggravate inflamed tendons. Floating and other gentle movements facilitate the healing of tendons.

PHYSICAL AND EMOTIONAL TRAUMA

All living beings are traumatized at some time. What is important is to minimize the number, intensity and effect of those we do face by protecting our body, mind, emotions and spirit from what Hamlet called "the thousand natural shocks that flesh is heir to." Defend yourself against traumatic intrusions, because severe trauma has altered, interrupted and even ended many productive lives.

HOW TO PROTECT YOURSELF FROM TRAUMA

MENTAL PROTECTION: Embody and generate harmony, peace and goodwill; indulge in affirmative, soothing, healing arts; envision affirmation, progress and serenity.

PHYSICAL PROTECTION: Feast on a bio-organic raw living food diet; enjoy consistent aerobic and resistance exercise; get proper and regular rest including sleep.

EMOTIONAL PROTECTION: Surround yourself with positive, loving people; share the best of yourself, and encourage others to do likewise; and affirm all the positive attributes of your life, then reaffirm them regularly.

SPIRITUAL PROTECTION: Contemplate, meditate or pray daily; be your best, and encourage others to be likewise; and nurture your unlimited universal essence.

ULCERS

Ulcers have become an irritant to people of every age. They usually occur in the stomach but can also be found in other parts of the body. The three primary causes of ulcers are stress (hectic schedules, family pressures, overwork, insufficient rest, especially sleep, and to little appropriate exercise); malnutrition (including overeating without substantive nutritional value); and infections, caused by such microbes as h-pylori. We can neutralize the occurrence and spread of ulcers by counteracting each of these causes:

REDUCE STRESS: Although, like trauma, stress is a part of life, just like trauma stress can be significantly reduced and sometimes eliminated.

COMBAT MALNUTRITION WITH HEALING FOODS: Broccoli, radishes and cabbage sprouts and their juices are powerful anti-ulcer agents. Sauerkraut, cabbage juice, cayenne pepper and garlic also calm and deter ulcers.

FIGHT MICROBIAL INFECTIONS: Use capsicum tincture, fenugreek extract, raw aloe vera, flaxseed water, osha, anti parasitic herbal supplements to avoid or reduce microbial infections.

URINARY TRACT PROBLEMS AND KIDNEY DYSFUNCTION

The flowing and filtering processes of the body are designed to be efficient; however, much of what goes through our bodies these days not only clogs those bodies but also causes them to be diseased. Kidney disorders and urinary tract infections are epidemic around the globe. Since they impede circulation and cardiovascular function, we must protect our organs of circulation and excretion.

PURE DIET: A healthy diet that includes plenty of pure liquids and excludes most proteins and fats promotes optimal renal and urinary tract functions. Eat and drink alkalizing foods of the raw vegan variety.

MEDICINAL SUPPLEMENTS: Cranberry seeds and their extract, grapefruit seed extract, probiotics, raw apple cider vinegar, lemon juice and lemon grass purge and empower the renal and urinary systems.

MASSAGE: Therapeutic bodywork helps alleviate swelling due to infection or edema; it also aids circulation, helping to remove impediments that can cause renal and urinary disorders.

ELECTROMAGNETIC THERAPY: This curative process is used extensively to reinvigorate the water-based organs of the body. The-non invasive techniques involved in electromagnetic therapy reestablish and intensify the proper functioning of these organs.

VARICOSE VEINS

As many of us, especially women, age we are distressed by these unnecessary and unsightly annoyances. Varicose veins are often caused by bad posture, an impacted colon or impaired circulation. The combination of one or several of these problems combined with excessive standing eventually causes varicose veins. Despite the severity and extent of this problem, you can combat or even eliminate it using the following means:

STRUCTURAL REALIGNMENT: Degenerative posture is a universal problem that worse more severe with age, so we must always try maintain our best posture. If necessary, consult an osteopathic or chiropractic practitioner.

COLON CLEANSING: A vegan diet and intestinal cleansing are two of the best ways to relax the muscles, nerves and veins of the lower extremities. Enemas and colonics — followed by implants of wheatgrass juice — are effective components of this process.

THERAPEUTIC INVERSION: Placing the lower body above the head by using a slant board promotes circulation and eases pressure on the lower extremities. Periodic inversion provides temporary relief from varicose veins; frequent therapeutic inversion eventually yields positive, permanent results.

OTHER THERAPIES: Modern medicine provides therapies using saline and lasers to reduce varicose veins; when they are properly administered, they reduce visible indication of varicose veins. Whirlpools, hot tubs and essential-oil baths also help reduce and eliminate these venous irritations.

WEIGHT PROBLEMS

Problems caused by excess weight plague those who live in so-called "advanced" societies where "food" is plentiful, but many also suffer from malnutrition — either self-imposed or imposed by society — that causes anorexia and other disorders.

SELF-RESPECT: Many of us use food to counteract pain, frustration, disappointment and stress. We eat too fast, too often and too casually, using food as a drug rather than as a nutritive resource. This is due primarily to a lack of self-respect: If we reclaim our self-regard, we can eat food appropriately instead of stuffing ourselves with non-nutritive excess.

DYNAMIC EXERCISE: When you want to reduce weight and/or increase muscle, become a dynamo at the gym rather than at the table. You can evaluate your progress by reshaping your body to its proper form as you increase strength and endurance. The beneficial results will motivate you to continue both aerobic and resistance training.

PSYCHOLOGICAL SELF-HEALING: With the assistance of a compassionate professional practitioner, you can make great progress in your weight regulation. Whether you want to modify your weight or stabilize it, the process of self-revelation, self-discovery and self-motivation in such therapy assists you in establishing and maintaining a trim and healthy body.

WEEKLY FASTING: The purpose of fasting is not to lose weight in a short time; instead, regular fasting incorporating raw juices and pure water cleanses body and spirit, providing the purification that leads to self-improvement of that body and that spirit.

YEAST INFECTIONS

This contemporary malady, which torments millions of people throughout the world, encompasses everything from mundane vaginal infections to the complex affliction known as candida. When our immune systems weaken as a result of unhealthy living, yeast assaults our bodies to become a permanent nemesis that creates constantly expanding fields of internal toxicity and pollution. The result is a biochemical imbalance that impedes the functions of every organ and of the entire physiological structure.

CONSTRUCTIVE DIET: Your anti-yeast diet should include raw vegetarian foods such as nuts, seeds, sprouted grains and beans, and raw vegetables from both sea and land. You must avoid all fruits, flour products, and condiments such as honey, sugar and maple syrup, because they provide the fuel which sustains the fungi that attack you.

THERAPEUTIC SOLUTIONS: Steam baths, Far-infrared saunas, ginger baths and sea-salt hot-water baths, hypothermia, hyperbarics, and other oxygen-based therapies help to purge the body of yeast.

SUPPLEMENTAL SOLUTIONS: Raw-garlic therapy, oregano oil, grapeseed and grapefruit-seed extract, and liquid O1 destroy fungi and yeast in the body.

SUNBATHING: Arrange your schedule and environment to accommodate sunbathing before 9 A.M. and after 4 P.M. in order to capture the indirect UV rays that help the immune system purge the body of unwanted yeast and fungi.

This also applies to those who care for children, other family members, and the infirm. (Please use the relevant parts of this book to guide you.)

CHAPTER FOURTEEN

CONTINUING CONTRIBUTION(S): FAMILY, FRIENDS AND COMMUNITY

One of the many blessings of longevity is the ability to continue to contribute. While many of us seek to reach retirement, we should, instead, seek to reach reinvigoration. That means that we do not put an arbitrary limit upon our service on behalf of ourselves and others. Self-respect creates the desire to give of ourselves, because we value ourselves enough to know that we have much to give. In fact, if we are fortunate enough to retire from formal established work, we can contribute more using our post-work accumulation of experience and wisdom. The unfortunate development of broken households affords us a unique and necessary opportunity to participate in the nurturing of families which are merely extensions of our own. In this instance, the maturity, wisdom and experience of accomplished longevity is an invaluable benefit. Contribution to others begins with the care and self-respect you bestow on yourself. This sustains and intensifies the three essential qualities of moral and ethical essence: focus, commitment and achievement. The gift of self is life-long. It starts with children caring for themselves, their siblings and pets and continues at every age. The accumulated experiences of sharing are its gift to continuing service during a rewarding longevity.

The gift of sharing oneself is cyclical. In maturity, you recall those who gave of themselves to you and your family and you will be gratified to be similarly remembered by those to whom you give of yourself. When you give freely of yourself, you not only do not lose any part, but instead, extend and increase the best aspects of who you are — while improving the lives that you serve. You achieve ever-increasing depth and dimension through service to others. This service is not limited to other people and to animals; it includes all of nature's environments which have given and continues to give so much to us. In our time, the environment badly needs our help and service. Every Sunday morning, our schedules permitting, my family and I walk along the shores of the Atlantic Ocean. Part of our routine has become the clearing of beach trash accumulated from industrial pollution, ocean-going vessels and the people who visit that beach. We have come to think of these walks as our time in church. The church is nature; the gospel is the wind; the tabernacle is the sky; and spiritual exhilaration is the result. At the end of each such pilgrimage, we stand for a moment looking at the ocean and give thanks for everything that is good and glorious in our lives. This mixture of natural and spiritual glory never fails to motivate me to give even more completely of myself in work, writing, and other contributions to the entire world.

This is life at its best and most simple: We give of ourselves to renew ourselves. We share to benefit others and, in the process, the sharing returns to us in inspiring ways.

A perfect example of self-fulfilling sharing is the creation of the Red Cross, begun in 1859 by a Swiss citizen, Henri Dunant. During his travels, he visited the Italian town of Solferino, where more than 40,000 people had died as a result of war. Trying to care for the more than 9,000 survivors, Dunant organized local citizens to bring the wounded into their homes and churches and public places to care for them. His efforts saved thousands of people and their families, and led Dunant to conclude that such assistance would continue to be necessary throughout the world. His dedication led him to write *A Memory of Solferino*, which became one of the most widely-read works of the 19th century. In it, he called for both governments and private citizens to create resources to help the casualties of war, and suggested a conference be held to establish an organization which could implement this idea.

This conference, held in Geneva on October 29, 1863, signaled the founding of the International Red Cross. Because of Dunant's efforts, the documents establishing the Geneva Convention were formalized. To this day, the sign of the Red Cross represents humanitarian assistance to everyone who needs it. Thousands of people have devoted their lives to the service of life: Confucius, Hippocrates, Saint Francis of Assisi, Louis Pasteur, Florence Nightingale, Clara Barton, Oscar Schindler, Raoul

Wallenberg, Mother Theresa, Jimmy Carter, the Dalai Lama, Desmond Tutu, Pele and Paul McCartney. All of us should strive to be a part of this distinguished group.

In *The Body Book*, Sara Stein explains that genetics is only partly responsible for successful longevity. She suggests that the unifying elements of fulfilling longevity are consistent happiness, contentment with one's work, acceptance of the inevitable and friendly interaction with others. These positive attitudes and behaviors enhance the body's life-sustaining chemistry by reducing the effects of stress hormones (especially cortisone), resulting in a stronger immune system.

A relaxed, calm person rarely secretes adrenaline, thus allowing the entire cardiovascular system to function fully and peacefully. Increased stress causes increased production of cortisone, which allows cholesterol-based hormones to bond, facilitating the likelihood of various dysfunctions including weight gain, irritability and liver problems.

The daughter of one of the leading families of Europe came to us at age 102 because she wanted to live another twenty years at full throttle. My first reaction was to ask her to teach us how to live more than 100 years so successfully. She replied, "Come to the gym tomorrow morning at 7, and I will teach you the exercises that have kept me limber and vital." Every person at The Institute, including guests and staff, was there on time. She ran us through an exhausting 90 minutes of exertion that would be too much for most youngsters. Then she said, "Now, you show me!" After a long and appropriate laugh, I responded, "You must continue as you have. I ask you only to stop thinking about age because, obviously, it is irrelevant to you." She thanked us and proceeded with her post-workout stretching. Her vital longevity continued until she was 107 year old.

Each of us must discover and pursue romance with life. And — as with all romance — the participants must share respect, reciprocal admiration and unified fulfillment. Since the essence of self-sharing is love, you must love yourself in order to give of yourself because you must consider yourself worthy of giving, and you must love others in order to truly give of yourself. When that love lasts a lifetime, you love your loving longevity.

CHAPTER FIFTEEN

AGELESS REALITY

Physics supports the reality of timelessness, because the scientific fact is that there is a time-space continuum; this means that when a given span of time appears to end, it is merely completing a cycle that is part of the complete unending entirety. Thus, the absolute reality is that our longevity not only survives us but takes us with it into the cyclical eternity.

"Physics" is a fascinatingly accurate word for this process because although our physical existence might have limits, our absolute continuity does not. The continuous contributions of many members of the human family validate the actuality of the enduring gifts eternity receives: The ideas and works of Carver, Cervantes, Curie, DaVinci, Einstein, Freud, Grieg, Gutenberg, Mandela, Meir, Moliere, Mozart, Schweitzer, Siddartha, Socrates, Strindberg, Tchaikovsky, and all the loving parents who give life and sustenance to every soul. Their gifts resonate throughout the ages, gracing time and space with wisdom, humanity and magnificence and filling our days with unlimited potential and fully realized grandeur.

Similarly, the art of your life should be a continuing example of caring, courtesy and culture, a distinguished tapestry of your best thoughts, finest acts and greatest contributions. An exuberant sharing of self elevates not only those who receive it but your own self as well, because the unending sequence of life is cyclical.

The ultimate reward is not to seek reward, but simply to know we have done and been our very best. Longevity is served by kindness, gentleness and excellence. Longevity — the word itself indicates that we must not be *short*-sighted, must not seek the immediate solution at the expense of long term problems. Why feed your body at the expense of robbing your soul? Why build a temporary dwelling by destroying a permanent ecology? Why consume self-destructively? Why lie, cheat and kill? Why excuse such excesses? Why not, instead, serve the continuous sphere of life wisely, naturally and harmoniously?

THE UNCHANGING TRUTHS

ATOMS: Appropriately, we start with atoms, which have been present from the beginning and are ever present. Everything is made of atoms. Atoms and their subatomic particles are at the core of every structure, human and otherwise. You must build every atom of your being through proper diet, exercise, rest and interaction.

BEAUTY: Despite the adage, beauty is not in the eye of the beholder; it is in the essence of the beheld. This means you must nourish your inner and outer beauty for every beholder, including you yourself, to gaze on with grateful wonder.

CHARITY: Another adage, this one true, is that charity begins at home. If you give yourself and your family your loving essence, that gift will eventually expand to include everyone and everything, eternally. Start your good works at home, and they will eventually benefit everyone everywhere.

DIVINITY: Like beauty, divinity is within each soul, to be honored by complete devotion to all that is good and sacred. When you live well and give completely, you serve your divine soul while it is part of your earthly self and thereafter.

ENLIGHTENMENT: Serving your divinity leads you to the light. When you are enlightened, you see, live and are everything that is virtuous, positive and life-affirming.

FLORA and FAUNA: They preceded humanity and dare us to sustain them. They represent the symbiotic biological harmony of ecology, for to nurture them is to sustain the essence of all life, including our own.

GRANDEUR: Appropriately, largesse is a significant part of grandeur. Grandeur is the ability to see, serve and live the greater good even if it appears to be a temporary detriment to our own progress. This demands the broad perspective rather than the petty imperative.

HARMONY: Like great music, life must be performed in harmony. Just as only cooperative interaction communicates the grandeur of a great symphony, we cannot conduct our lives to the constant irritation of disharmony. Harmony must begin within each of us in order to extend to all of us.

INSIGHT: As we negotiate the journey of life, we must see beyond, behind and beneath each individual path in order to perceive the purpose of the entire voyage and its ultimate destination. Fulfilled longevity develops insight, and insight informs purposeful longevity, just as knowledge and understanding promote peace, progress, potential and purpose. As Socrates said, the unexamined life is not worth living.

JOY: Every minute must be lived with profound joy. Joy must be a part of waking, sleeping, lovemaking, art. Abundant joy will always find its way to others and back to its source. The joyous life celebrates and fills longevity with exhilaration.

KINDNESS: Kindness is sympathy and empathy in action. When we feel for and with others, we treat them with open hearts and helping hands. Like joy, kindness goes from us only to be returned in kind.

LIFE: Pedro Calderon de la Barca wrote the play *La Vida Es Sueno* (*Life Is a Dream*). We must make life a glorious daily dream not only for ourselves but for every dreamer. Embracing the dream, we live the dream.

MOTION: Newton's First Law of Gravity: "An entity at rest tends to stay at rest; an entity in motion tends to stay in motion." A living entity must do both, but when you are in motion it should always be constructive and progressive motion. Do nothing that will impede your own progress or anyone else's.

NOBILITY: Nobility is not the exclusive province of royalty but the birthright of every soul. Your essential nobility demands that you live in harmony with every soul, including your own spirit.

OPTIMISM: The word optimism comes from the Latin root "opti," meaning "best." The best attitude is one of optimism, for to anticipate the best is to assure the best. (Always opt for optimism!)

PURPOSE: Many people spend their lives wondering about the purpose of life and their place in that purpose. John Wesley provided the answers in his Rules:

> *Do all the good you can,*
> *By all the means you can,*
> *In all the ways you can,*
> *In all the places you can,*
> *At all the times you can,*
> *To all the people you can,*
> *As long as ever you can.*

QUINTESSENCE: Just as atoms have subatomic particles, the essence of essence is quintessence. When we seek to answer philosophical questions, we are trying to determine the quintessence of existence, a quintessence that is superbly defined by one word: Love!

RENAISSANCE: Although part of our history is called "the Renaissance," the literal rebirth of our cells is an ongoing phenomenon. Because we continuously regenerate ourselves, these never-ending rebirths give us the opportunity to grow, expand and change as we literally recreate ourselves.

SIMPLICITY: The essential simplicity of all goodness is aptly expressed in the phrase, "First, do no harm." It really is that simple: Hurt no life, including your own.

TRANQUILITY: The Sea of Tranquility is on the moon, but the limitless reality of tranquility is in the soul. Your sense of peace is crucial to healthy longevity. Again, your tranquility touches others and is returned to you intensified. Which means the cliché, "Peace of mind," like most clichés, is true.

UNITY: When we discussed harmony, we focused upon mutually beneficial interaction with others. Unity is the integrated totality of the self, the internal harmony of each given soul. But there is a critical connection between harmony and unity; unity means oneness, and you must be a unified self to achieve complete harmony with others.

VISION: Both unity and harmony require the comprehensive vision to see the totality: We must see the big picture and not focus on confusing details. Remember another valid cliché: "None is so blind as he who will not see."

WISDOM: Wisdom is one of the many rewards of insightful longevity. The maturity provided by accumulated knowledge, understanding, compassion and emotional stability makes us wise, and it is only wisdom that can guide us appropriately.

X=X: THE GREAT UNKNOWN: One of the most important benefits of properly cultivated longevity is the ability to know what must be known but once seemed undecipherable. So the X that, in mathematical formations, represents the unknown is replaced by understanding in the mind of responsible adults. You have the answers. And they are all positive.

YIN/YANG: Our disparate elements seek balance; the yin and the yang must interact harmoniously to stabilize us. Ancient cultures developed their philosophies on the foundation of this profound truth, and we need to function similarly, seeking to restore both the internal and external equilibrium that have been sabotaged by our anti-natural inclinations.

ZEN: Just as we began appropriately with the all-informing atom, we end appropriately with the all-encompassing Zen. Zen knows no limits of language, geography, history or tradition. It is the universal totality we seek, only to discover that it has always been a part of us just as we have always been a part of it. Zen is the quintessence of life: The good, simple, whole essence of being, infinite and eternal. Quintessential realities embody the core of life. Without them you are lost; with them, you are complete. These are not mere concepts, but quite the opposite: They are the building-blocks of the life well-lived, of the longevity properly served.

Rediscover and respect these eternal cornerstones of understanding; they will constitute the foundations of the grandest dwelling of your complete longevity.

CHAPTER SIXTEEN

CONCLUSION:
LIVING LEGACY

The journey of life is not unlike our journey through this book. We make discoveries that make each step forward a joyous surprise as well as a continuing celebration. As we progress, we assure that our legacy will be constantly beneficial and fondly remembered. In *As You Like It*, William Shakespeare chronicles the conventionally held negative process of life in a speech that has become so famous that it has its own title: "The Seven Ages of Man."

> All the world's a stage,
> And all the men and women merely players;
> They have their exits and their entrances,
> And one man in his time plays many parts,
> His acts being seven ages. At first, the infant,
> Mewling and puking in the nurse's arms.
> Then the whining schoolboy with his satchel
> And shining morning face, creeping like snail
> Unwillingly to school. And then the lover
> Sighing like furnace, with a woeful ballad
> Made to his mistress' eyebrow. Then a soldier,
> Full of strange oaths, and bearded like the pard,
> Jealous in honour, sudden and quick to quarrel,
> Seeking the bubble reputation
> Even in the cannon's mouth. And then the justice,
> In fair round belly with good capon lin'd,
> With eyes severe and beard of formal cut,
> Full of wise saws and modern instances;
> And so he plays his part. The sixth age shifts

Into the lean and slipper'd pantaloon,
With spectacles on nose, and pouch on side;
His youthful hose well sav'd, a world too wide
For his shrunk shank, and his big manly voice,
Turning again toward childish treble, pipes
And whistles in his sound. Last scene of all,
That ends this strange eventful history,
Is second childishness and mere oblivion,
Sans teeth, sans eyes, sans taste, sans everything.

Even Shakespeare, brilliant as he was and as the speech is, could be wrong. His representation of life is ironic, amusing, bittersweet — and shortsighted. He was not privy to the benefits life now provides to mature fulfillment. His description of life's later stages reflects a world we can easily change, and the later stages can, for us, be more gratifying than the best times of previous generations. All that is necessary for fulfilling longevity is the committed flexibility of vision, dedication and purpose that requires us to appreciate life at every stage.

There are benefits to our understanding that life is a cycle that must end; among those benefits is the desire to fill the given time lovingly, passionately and completely. Another is the compelling opportunity to reflect about the legacy we wish to leave. This reality compels us to ask the question "What kind of legacy do I want to leave? Do I want to be remembered as a petty, greedy, unyielding, abusive vacuum? Or is my permanent testament one of love, kindness, humanity, sharing, and integrity?" The answer is obvious. And the means to achieving it — to living it — are readily available: The Longevity Program.

SELECTED BIBLIOGRAPHY

The number of books, manuals, pamphlets, articles, essays, studies and Internet items about longevity is as limitless as healthy longevity itself, especially in our technological age. This selected bibliography reflects the most crucial and comprehensive aspects of The Longevity Program and the wasteful and harmful modes of anti-life procedures.

Neither the author of this book, individually or together, nor The Hippocrates Health Institute nor any of its functionaries endorses the authors, theories or content of any cited sources unless specifically stated.

BOOKS

Arnot, Robert, M.D. *Dr. Bob Arnot's Guide to Turning Back the Clock.* Boston: Little, Brown and Company, 1995.

Bach, Edward, M.D. and E. J. Wheeler, M.D. *The Bach Flower Remedies.* New Canaan, CT: Keats Publishing, 1979.

Barnard, Neal, M.D. *Food for Life: How the New Four Food Groups Can Save Your Life.* New York: Harmony Books, 1993.

Bergner, Paul. *The Healing Power of Echinacea and Goldenseal and Other Immune System Herbs.* Rocklin, CA: Prima Publishing, 1997.

Berwick, Ann. *Holistic Aromatherapy: Balance the Body and the Soul with Essential Oils.* St. Paul, MN: Llwellyn Publications, 1994.

Bernay-Roman, Andy. *Deep Feeling, Deep Healing: The Heart, Mind, and Soul of Getting Well.* Jupiter, FL: Spectrum Healing Press, 2001.

Bloomfield, Harold H., M.D. and Robert B. Kory. *The Holistic Way to Health and Happiness: A New Approach to Complete Lifetime Wellness.* New York: Fireside, 1978.

Blum, Deborah. *Sex on the Brain: The Biological Differences Between Men and Women.* New York: Viking, 1997.

Bolles, Edmund Blair. *Remembering and Forgetting: Inquiries into the Nature of Memory.* New York: Walker and Company, 1988.

Bonar, Ann. *Herbs: A Complete Guide to Their Cultivation.* London: Tiger Books International, 1992.

Bragdon, Allen D. and David Gamon, Ph.D. *Brains That Work a Little Bit Differently: Recent Discoveries About Common Brain Diversities.* New York: Barnes & Noble Books, 2000.

Brody, Jane. *Jane Brody's Nutrition Book: A Lifetime Guide to Good Eating for Better Health and Weight Control*. New York: W. W. Norton & Company, 1981.

Campbell, Don. *The Mozart Effect: Tapping the Power of Music to Heal the Body, Strengthen the Mind and Unlock the Creative Spirit*. New York: Avon Books, 1997.

Carper, Jean. *Food — Your Miracle Medicine: How Food Can Prevent and Cure over 100 Symptoms and Problems*. New York: HarperCollins, 1993.

Castleman, Michael. *The Healing Herbs: The Ultimate Guide to the Curative Power of Nature's Medicines*. Emmaus, PA: Rodale Press, 1991.

Chen, Ze-lin, M.D. and Chen, Mei-fang, M.D. *A Comprehensive Guide to Chinese Herbal Medicine*. Edison, NJ: Castle Books, 1999.

Chopra, Deepak, M.D. *Ageless Body, Timeless Mind: The Quantum Alternative to Growing Old*. New York: Harmony Books, 1993.

Chopra, Deepak, M.D. *Creating Health: Beyond Prevention, Toward Perfection*. Boston: Houghton Mifflin Company, 1987.

Christopher, John R., Dr. *School of Natural Healing*. Provo, Utah: BiWorld Publishers, 1976.

Claflin, Edward (Editor). *Healing Yourself with Food (Prevention's System of Health and Natural Healing)*. Emmaus, PA: Rodale Press, 1995.

Clement, Brian R. *Belief: All There Is . . .* West Palm Beach, FL: Hippocrates Publications, 1991.

Clement, Brian R. *Croyances*. Quebec: Les Editions Trustar, 1996.

Clement, Brian R. *Exercise: Creating Your Persona*. West Palm Beach, FL: A M Press, 1994.

Clement, Brian R. *Hippocrates Health Program: A Proven Guide to Healthful Living*. West Palm Beach, FL: Hippocrates Publications, 1989.

Clement, Brian R. *Living Foods for Optimum Health: Staying Healthy in an Unhealthy World*. Roseville, CA: Prima Publishing, 1998.

Clement, Brian R and Anna Maria. *Relationships: Voyages Through Life*. West Palm Beach, FL: A.M. Press, 1994.

Clement, Brian R. *Spirituality in Healing and Life*. West Palm Beach, FL: Hippocrates Publications, 1997.

Colgrove, Melba, Ph.D., Harold H. Bloomfield, M.D. and Peter McWilliams. *How to Survive the Loss of a Love*. Los Angeles: Prelude Press, 1991.

Cox, Peter. *You Don't Need Meat*. New York: Thomas Dunne Books, 2002.

Dalai Lama and Howard C. Cutler, M.D. *The Art of Happiness: A Handbook for Living*. New York: Riverhead Books, 1998.

Deacon, Terrence W. *The Symbolic Species: The Co-Evolution of Language and the Brain*. New York: W. W. Norton, 1997.

Dharma Singh Khalsa, M.D. with Cameron Stauth. *Brain Longevity: The Breakthrough Medical Program that Improves Your Mind and Memory*. New York: Warner Books, 1997.

Diamond, Harvey and Marilyn. *Fit for Life: The natural body cycle, permanent weight loss plan that proves it's not "what" you eat, but when and how!* New York: Warner Books, 1985.

Diamond, Harvey. *Fit for Life: A New Beginning*. New York: Kensington Books, 2000.

Dodt, Colleen K. *The Essential Oils Book: Creating Personal Blends for Mind & Body*. Pownal, VT: Storey Communications, 1996.

Dollemore, Doug, Mark Giuliucci and the Editors of Men's Health Magazine. *Age Erasers for Men: Hundreds of Fast and Easy Ways to Beat the Years*. Emmaus, PA: Rodale Press, 1994.

Dossey, Larry, M.D. *Healing Words: The Power of Prayer and the Practice of Medicine*. San Francisco: HarperSanFrancisco, 1993.

Duke, James A., Ph.D. *Dr. Duke's Essential Herbs: 13 Vital Herbs You Need to Disease-Proof Your Body, Boost Your Energy, Lengthen Your Life*. Emmaus, PA: Rodale, 1999.

Evans, Mark. *Natural Home Remedies: Safe, Effective and Traditional Treatments for Common Ailments*. New York: Anness Publishing, 1996.

Farmilant, Eunice. *The Natural Foods Sweet Tooth Cookbook*. New York: Pyramid Books, 1975.

Finley, Anita & Bill. *Live to be 100 Plus: Chart Your Way to a Longer Life*. Boca Raton, FL: Senior Life Press, 1992.

Fischer Rizzi, Susanne. *Medicine of the Earth: Legends, Recipes, and Cultivation of Healing Plants*. Portland, OR: Rudra Press, 1996.

Forni, P. M. *Choosing Civility: The Twenty-five Rules of Considerate Conduct*. New York: St. Martin's Press, 2002.

Foster, Steven. *101 Medicinal Herbs: An Illustrated Guide*. Loveland, CO: Interweave Press, 1998.

Fraser, Linda. *Classic Vegetarian Cooking.* London: Barnes & Noble Books, 2001.

Fuhrman, Joel, M.D. *Eat to Live: The Revolutionary Formula for Fast and Sustained Weight Loss.* Boston: Little, Brown and Company, 2003.

Goleman, Daniel, Ph.D. *Emotional Intelligence: Why It Can Matter More Than IQ.* New York: Bantam Books, 1995.

Glynn, Ian. *An Anatomy of Thought: The Origin and Machinery of the Mind.* New York: Oxford University Press, 1999.

Gosselin, Robert E., M.D., Harold C. Hodge, Roger P. Smith, and Marion N. Gleason. *Clinical Toxicology of Commercial Products.* Baltimore: The Williams & Wilkins Co., 1977.

Haas, Robert. *Eat to Win: The Sports Nutrition Bible.* New York: Signet, 1983.

Haas, Robert. *Permanent Remissions: Life-Extending Diet Strategies That Can Help Prevent and Reverse Cancer, Heart Disease, Diabetes, and Osteoporosis.* New York: Pocket Books, 1997.

Haber, David. *Health Promotion and Aging: Implications for the Health Professions.* New York: Springer Publishing Company, 1999.

Hill, Napoleon and Michael J. Ritt, Jr. *Napoleon Hill's Keys to Positive Thinking: 10 Steps to Health, Wealth and Success.* New York: Dutton, 1998.

Hobson, J. Allan, M.D. *The Chemistry of Conscious States: How the Brain Changes Its Mind.* New York: Little, Brown and Company, 1994.

Hogshead, Nancy and Gerald Secor Couzens. *Asthma and Exercise.* New York: Henry Holt and Company, 1990.

Holford, Patrick and Dr. Hyla Kass. *Natural Highs: Increase Your Energy; Sharpen Your Mind; Improve Your Mood; Relax and Beat Stress with Legal Natural and Healthy Mind-Altering Substances.* London: Judy Piatkus Publishers, 2001.

Howard, Pierce J., Ph.D. *The Owner's Manual for the Brain: Everyday Applications from Mind-Brain Research.* Austin, TX: Leornian Press, 1994.

Hutton, Ginger. *Reflections — Thoughts on Love and Living.* Phoenix: The Arizona Republic, 1980.

Jensen, Bernard, M.D. *Dr. Jensen's Juicing Therapy: Nature's Way to Better Health and a Longer Life.* Los Angeles: Keats Publishing, 2000.

Johnson, G. Timothy, Editor. *The Harvard Medical School health letter book.* Cambridge, MA: Harvard University Press, 1981.

Jonas, Wayne B., M.D. and Jennifer Jacobs, M.D. *Healing with Homeopathy: The Complete Guide.* New York: Warner Books, 1996.

Kiley, Dan, Dr. *The Peter Pan Syndrome: Men Who Have Never Grown Up.* New York: Avon Books, 1983.

Ledoux, Joseph. *The Emotional Brain: The Mysterious Underpinnings of Emotional Life.* New York: Touchstone, 1996.

Lerner, Harriet, Ph.D. *The Dance of Anger: A Woman's Guide to Changing the Patterns of Intimate Relationships.* New York: Perennial Library, 1989.

Levine, Stephen. *Healing into Life and Death.* New York: Anchor Books, 1977.

Life Extension Foundation. *Disease Prevention and Treatment.* Hollywood, FL: Life Extension Media, 2003.

Linkletter, Art. *Old Age Is Not for Sissies: Choices for Senior Americans.* New York: Viking Penguin, Inc., 1988.

Lipschitz, David A., M.D., Ph.D., *Breaking the Rules of Aging.* Washington, D. C.: Lifeline Press, 2002.

Little, Paul E. *Know Why You Believe.* Wheaton IL: Victor Books, 1973.

Lockie, Andrew, M.D. and Nicola Geddes, M.D. *Complete Guide to Homeopathy: The Principles and Practice of Treatment..* New York: DK Publishing, 2000.

Lockie, Andrew, M.D. and Nicola Geddes, M.D. *Homeopathy: The Principles and Practice of Treatment.* New York: DK Publishing, 1995.

Lowe, Carl, James W. Nechas, and the editors of Prevention Magazine. *Whole Body Healing: Natural Healing with Movement, Exercise, Massage and Other Drug-Free Methods.* Emmaus, PA: Rodale Press, 1983.

Maimonides: *Medical Writings (A Series, Translated and Annotated by Fred Rosner, M.D.)* Haifa: The Maimonides Research Institute, 1988.

Mamonov, Valery, Ph.D. *Control for Life Extension: A Personalized Holistic Approach.* Rome, ME: Long Life Press, 2001.

Marshall, John, M.D. with Heather Barbash. *The Sports Doctor's Fitness Book for Women.* New York: Delacorte Press, 1981.

McCabe, Vinton. *Homeopathy, Healing and You.* New York: St. Martin's Griffin, 1999.

McCabe, Vinton. *Practical Homeopathy.* New York: St. Martin's Griffin, 2000.

Men's Health Magazine. *The Men's Health Longevity Program.* Emmaus, PA: Rodale Press, 2001.

Messina, Virginia and Mark Messina. *The Vegetarian Way: Total Health for You and Your Family.* New York: Crown, 1996.

Mindell, Earl R. *Earl Mindell's Food as Medicine: What You Can Eat to Help Prevent Everything From Colds to Heart Disease to Cancer.* New York: Fireside (Simon & Schuster), 1994.

Navarra, Tova and Myron A. Lipkowitz. *Encyclopedia of Vitamins, Minerals and Supplements.* New York: Facts on File, 1996.

Naylor, Nicola. *Discover Essential Oils (First-Step Handbook to Better Health).* Berkeley, CA: Ulysses Press, 1998.

Nirenberg, Jesse S., Ph.D. *Getting Through to People.* Engelwood Cliffs, NJ: Prentice Hall, 1963.

Northrup, Christiane, M.D. *Women's Bodies, Women's Wisdom.* New York: Bantam Books, 1998.

Ohno, Yoshitaka, M.D., Ph.D. *A Guide to Achieving Better Health and Aging.* Willoughby, OH: Ohno Institute on Water and Health (Undated).

Passwater, Richard A., Ph.D. *The Longevity Factor: Chromium Picolinate.* New Canaan, CT: Keats Publishing, 1993.

Peck, M. Scott, M.D. *The Road Less Traveled: A New Psychology of Love, Traditional Values and Spiritual Growth.* New York: Touchstone, 1978.

Peikin, Steven R., M.D. *The Feel Full Diet: The Medically Proven, Nutritionally Sound Weight Loss Program that Stimulates the Release of Your Secret Anti-Hunger Mechanism.* New York: Atheneum, 1987.

Doctor's Little Black Bag of Remedies and Cures. Boardroom Inc., 1999.

Pritikin, Nathan. *Pritikin Permanent Weight-Loss Manual.* New York: Grosset & Dunlap, 1981.

Rath, Matthias, M.D. *Why Animals Don't Get Heart Attacks but People Do.* Fremont, CA: MR Publishing, 2003.

Ratey, John J., M.D. *A User's Guide to the Brain: Perception, Attention, and the Four Theaters of the Brain.* New York: Vintage Books, 2001.

Reich, Charles A. *The Greening of America.* New York: Random House, 1970.

Reid, Daniel P. *Chinese Herbal Medicine.* Boston: Shambhala Publications, 1999.

Reid, Daniel P. *The Complete Book of Chinese Health*. Boston: Shambhala Publications, 1994.

Reinhard, Tonia. *The Vitamin Sourcebook*. Los Angeles: Lowell House, 1998.

Restak, Richard, M.D. *Mozart's Brain and the Fighter Pilot: Unleashing Your Brain's Potential*. New York: Harmony Books, 2001.

Reuben, David R., M.D. *Everything You Always Wanted to Know about Nutrition*. New York: Avon Books, 1978.

Rister, Robert. *Japanese Herbal Medicine: The Healing Art of Kampo*. Garden City Park, NY: Avery Publishing Group, 1999.

Robertson, Ian H. *Mind Sculpture: Unlocking Your Brain's Untapped Potential*. New York: Fromm International, 2000.

Robbins, John. *Diet for a New America: How Your Food Choices Affect Your Health, Happiness and the Future of Life on Earth*. Walpole, NH: Stillpoint Publishing, 1987.

Robbins, John. *Reclaiming Our Health: Exploding the Medical Myth and Embracing the Source of True Healing*. Tiburon, CA: H J Kramer, 1996.

Robbins, William. *The American Food Scandal: Why You Can't Eat Well on What You Earn*. New York: William Morrow & Company, 1974.

Rondberg, Terry A., D.C. *Chiropractic First: The Fastest Growing Healthcare Choice Before Drugs or Surgery*. Chandler, AZ: The Chiropractic Journal, 1996.

Rose, Barry, M.D. and Christina Scott Moncrief, M.D. *Homeopathy for Women: A Comprehensive, Easy-to-Use Guide for Women of All Ages*. London: Collins & Brown, 1998.

Rosenfeld, Isadore, M.D. *The Complete Medical Exam*. New York: Avon Books, 1978.

Rosner, Fred, M.D. *Maimonides: Medical Writings (a series)*. Haifa, Israel: The Maimonides Research Institute, 1984 ongoing.

Schnaubelt, Kurt. *Medical Aromatherapy: Healing with Essential Oils*. Berkeley, CA: Frog, Ltd., 1999.

Schiller, Carol and David Schiller. *500 Formulas for Aromatherapy: Mixing Essential Oils for Every Use*. New York, NY: Sterling Publishing, 1994.

Sears, Barry (with Bill Lawren). *Enter the Zone: The Dietary Road Map to Lose Weight and More*. New York: Regan Books — HarperCollins, 1995.

Segal, Jeanne S., Ph.D. *Raising Your Emotional Intelligence: A Practical Guide*. New York: Henry Holt and Company, 1997.

Serrentino, Joe. *How Natural Remedies Work: Vitamins, Minerals, Nutrients, Homeopathic and Naturopathic Remedies*. Point Roberts, WA: Hartley & Marks, 1991.

Shankle, William Rodman, M.S., M.D. and Daniel G Amen, M.D. *Preventing Alzheimer's: Ways to Help Prevent, Delay, Detect, and Even Halt Alzheimer's Disease and Other Forms of Memory Loss*. New York: G. P. Putnam's Sons, 2004.

Siegel, Bernie S., M.D. *Love, Medicine and Miracles: Lessons Learned about Self-Healing from a Surgeon's Experience with Exceptional Patients*. New York: Harper & Row, 1987.

Simonton, O. Carl, M.D., Stephanie Mathews Simonton, James L. Creighton. *Getting Well Again: The Bestselling Classic About the Simontons' Revolutionary Lifesaving Self-Awareness Techniques*. New York: Bantam Books, 1992.

Smith, Jeffrey M. *Seeds of Deception: Exposing Industry and Government Lies About the Safety of the Genetically Engineered Foods You're Eating*. Fairfield, Iowa: Yes! Books, 2003.

Snow, Kimberly. *In Buddha's Kitchen: Cooking, Being Cooked and Other Adventures at a Meditation Center*. Boston: Shambhala Publications, 2003.

Staudacher, Carol. *Men and Grief: A Guide for Men Surviving the Death of a Loved One*. Oakland, CA: New Harbinger Publications, 1991.

Steiner, Claude, Ph.D. with Paul Perry. *Achieving Emotional Literacy: A Personal Program to Increase Your Emotional Intelligence*. New York: Avon Books, 1997.

Stillerman, Elaine, L.M.T. *The Encyclopedia of Bodywork: From Acupressure to Zone Therapy*. New York: Facts on File, 1996.

Stone, Irwin. *The healing factor: "vitamin C" against disease*. New York: Grosset & Dunlap, 1972.

Thayer, Robert E., Ph.D. *The Origin of Everyday Moods: Managing Energy, Tension, and Stress*. New York: Oxford University Press, 1996.

Thomas, Peggy. *Medicines from Nature*. New York, NY: Twenty First Century Books, 1997.

Tisserand, Robert B. *The Art of Aromatherapy: The Healing and Beautifying Properties of the Essential Oils of Flowers and Herbs*. Rochester, VT: Healing Arts Press, 1977.

Ursell, Amanda. *Vitamins and Minerals Handbook*. New York: Dorling Kindersley, 2001.

Varner, Sam, CSCS. *Slimmer, Younger, Stronger: 12 Simple Things You Can Do to Achieve Optimum Health*. Boston: Element, 2000.

Vertosick, Frank T. *When the Air Hits Your Brain: Tales of Neurosurgery*. New York: W. W. Norton and Company, 1996.

Walker, N. W., M.D., D.Sc. *The Vegetarian Guide to Diet & Salad*. Phoenix, AZ: Norwalk Press, 1986.

Weber, George, Ph.D. *Protecting Your Health with Probiotics — The "Friendly" Bacteria*. Green Bay, WI: IMPAKT Communications, 2001.

PERIODICALS

Please note that no original page listings are provided for these periodicals because in this cyber age publications are readily available and often accessible online, where they are often configured in various non-traditional formats, some of which omit or alter conventional pagination.

"Alzheimer's may begin at younger age." *The Palm Beach Post*, December 16, 2003.

Berreby, David. "Evolving by accident, not fitness." *The New York Times*, December 31, 2003.

"Better Brains: How Neuroscience Will Enhance You." *Scientific American*, Special Issue, September, 2003.

"Building a Better Grain: Studying Carotenoids in Rice and Corn." *Folio*, Fall, 2003.

"Cancer research yields clues to graying hair: The unsightly sign of aging provides insights about melanoma." The Associated Press, December 24, 2004.

Carson, Ben, M.D. "Your Mind Can Map Your Destiny." *Parade*, December 7, 2003.

Castleman, Michael. "Power Plants: The 10 best herbs for what ails you." *Modern Maturity*, January/February 2003.

"Chinese herbal drug in demand to battle malaria." *New York Times*, May 10, 2004.

Condon, Garrett. "Diet of fruits and vegetables lowers health costs." *The Hartford Courant*, June 22, 2003.

"Demand for obesity surgery grows worldwide." The Associated Press, May 30, 2004.

Dresbach, Sereana Howard and Amy Rossi. "Phytochemicals — Vitamins of the Future?" Ohio State University Extension Fact Sheet (HYG 5050 98)

"Driving more gives obesity a fat chance." The Associated Press, May 31, 2004.

"Emotional distress may speed aging of body's cells, study says," *The New York Times*, Tuesday, November 30, 2004.

"Epidemic of obesity spanning globe." The Associated Press, May 9, 2004.

"Exercise appears to aid breast cancer recovery." The Associated Press, March 30, 2004.

"Fat cells toxic to body, researchers find." The Associated Press, May 11, 2004.

Fields, R. Douglas. "The Other Half of the Brain: Mounting evidence suggests that glial cells, overlooked for half a century, may be nearly as critical to thinking and learning as neurons are." *Scientific American*, April, 2004.

"Folate may cut heart disease, stroke deaths." The Associated Press, March 6, 2004.

"Genetically modified food backed: The U. N. says farmer should grow food crops, not cash crops." *Los Angeles Times*, May 18, 2004.

"Global health ministers agree to urge sugar intake limit: The move is part of a plan to fight worldwide obesity." The Associated Press, May 22, 2004.

Gorman, Christine. "The No. 1 Killer of Women: No, it's not breast cancer. More women die of heart disease than of all cancers combined." *Time*, April 28, 2003.

"The Happiness Equation." *Smithsonian Magazine*, May 6, 2004.

Harrison, Don. "It's No day at the Beach: Worldwide, 70 percent of our beaches are eroding. Pollution and shoreline overdevelopment compound the problem." *Parade*, June 6, 2004.

"Health organizations want poultry in Asia to be vaccinated." *The New York Times*, February 6, 2004.

Hendricks, Melissa. "Keeping the Beat: These new heart tests could save your life." *AARP The Magazine*, March/April 2004.

"How Your Love Life Keeps You Healthy." *Time*, Special Issue, January 19, 2004.

"How to Save the Earth." *Time*, Special Report, August 26, 2002.

Jetter, Alexis. "How Safe Is Your Food?: One fish, two fish, red snapper, swordfish: A Menace Lurks in Your 'Healthy' Meal." *Reader's Digest*, August, 2003.

Kirchheimer, Sid. "Health report: Extra! Extra! Read all about the essential vitamins and minerals you need now — and where to get them." *AARP The Magazine*, January/February 2004.

Lee, Renee C. "Fatigue, insomnia may signal heart attack." The Associated Press, November 4, 2003.

Leith, Scott. "India upset over reports of pesticides in Coke, Pepsi." *The Palm Beach Post*, August 17, 2003.

Leonhardt, David. "U. S. Europe food dispute sprouts anew: Discussions about genetically modified food break down." *The New York Times*, June 20, 2003.

"Losing just a little weight can benefit the health of the obese." The Associated Press, May 31, 2004.

"Low drinking can harm brain tissue." The Associated Press, December 5, 2003.

"Low tar cigarettes no less hazardous, study finds." The Associated Press, January 9, 2004.

"Lung cancer in women an epidemic, report says." *Newsday*. April 14, 2004.

Mirsky, Steve. "Aroma Therapy." *Scientific American*, February, 2004.

Moffat, Anne. "Gumming Up Your Heart: Better Dental Care Can Prevent Disease and Keep You Healthier from Head to Toe." *AARP Bulletin*, March, 2004.

Nesmith, Jeff. "Polluted air may increase pollen: Experts see link between carbon dioxide, asthma." *Palm Beach Post Cox News Service*. May 1 2004.

Nesmith, Jeff. "Study links Alzheimer's to diabetes: Those with diabetes were 65 percent more likely to get Alzheimer's." *Palm Beach Post Cox News Service*. May 18, 2004.

"New research diminishes role of good cholesterol." *The New York Times*, March 15, 2004.

"Nutrition shortage hurting nations' mental capacities." The Associated Press, March 25, 2004.

"Obesity may affect some women's pay." The Associated Press, March 4, 2004.

"Obesity soon likely to kill more people than smoking." *The Washington Post*, March 10, 2004.

Oz, Mehmet, M.D. "Healing with an Open Mind: A surgeon learns to trust the wisdom of other medical traditions." *Parade*, November 30, 2003.

"Healthy Minds, Healthy Bodies: A Special Issue." *Parade*, October 12, 2003.

"Some fear bottled water draining Earth's supply." The Associated Press, June 8, 2003.

Thomas, Wiliam H., M.D. "The Search for Being: Why Making the Shift from Adult to Elder Is Not an Easy Passage," *AARP Bulletin*, November, 2004.

Stein, Bob. "Desire to eat fattening food tied to chronic stress." *The Washington Post*, September 30, 2003.

Stein, Bob. "Study links heavy use of antibiotics, breast cancer." *The Washington Post*, February 17, 2004.

"Study: Even older mice extend life by eating less." The Associated Press, March 25, 2004.

"Study links diet rich in seafood, red meat to gout." The Associated Press, March 11, 2004.

"Study links fat to 90,000 U. S. cancer deaths a year." The Associated Press, April 24, 2003.

"Study: Same brain site logs heartache, pain." The Associated Press, October 10, 2003.

"Study warns of salmon risks: Farm raised fish had higher pollutants." The Associated Press, January 9, 2004.

Susman, Carolyn. "Sleepless see health go astray." *The Palm Beach Post*, October 2, 2003.

Susman, Carolyn. "Study reveals stronger link between diabetes, heart disease." *The Palm Beach Post*, April 28, 2004.

Tanner, Lindsey. "Light exercise found to halt weight gain." The Associated Press, January 13, 2004.

"Ultrahigh dose chemotherapy of little good for breast cancer." The Associated Press, July 3, 2003.

"Vegetarian diet lowers cholesterol without pills." *The Palm Beach Post*, October 29, 2003.

"Women eating more calories, especially carbs." The Associated Press, February 6, 2004.

(Please note: Faults in grammar, syntax, capitalization, punctuation et al., and presumably unintended puns in any of the cited sources merely replicate the originals.)

Index

Nutriceuticals 29
Nuts 35, 39, 40, 45, 48, 71, 108, 114, 142, 157

O

Oats 98, 124
Onion 61, 112
Optimism 127, 166
Orally 65, 116, 117, 137
Oregano 40, 158
Ornish 118
Oxford University Press 46, 176, 180
Oxygen 23, 27, 28, 36, 41, 42, 44, 45, 47, 54, 68, 82, 95, 99, 109, 111, 113, 120, 135, 136, 138, 148, 150, 157

P

Papaya 48
Parkinson's disease 67, 83, 145
Parsley 48, 108
Parsnip 48, 144
Pea 35, 48, 61, 98
Peaches 48
Pears 48
Pecans 35, 40, 48
Pennsylvania College 112
Ph. 3, 9, 46, 121, 140, 173, 174, 175, 176, 177, 178, 180, 181
Phlebitis 66, 110, 123, 146
Phospholipids 32, 33, 35
Phytochemicals 28, 47, 54, 182
Phytonutrients 45, 98
Pilates 74
Pincemail 40
Pineapple 86
Pineapples 134
Prostate 62, 64, 66, 94, 96, 147
Protein 27, 32, 54, 61, 62, 63, 82, 98, 108, 118, 142, 152
Proteins 32, 35, 46, 47, 53, 63, 64, 65, 98, 118, 128, 141, 142, 155

Psoriasis 148
Pumpkin 34, 48, 147

Q

Quinoa 38, 62

R

Radicchio 48, 98
Radish 59
Resistance exercise 24, 58, 74, 75, 92, 129, 139, 142, 144, 154
Rheumatism 74, 111
Roberts 38, 180
Root vegetable 60, 62, 97
Root-vegetable 48
Rosemary 48
Rueff 38
Rush University 103
Rutabaga 48, 62, 112, 132

S

Sage 48
Salk Institute 103
Sapolsky 44
Scientific American 21, 181, 182, 183
Serotonin 31, 32, 36, 64, 128
Sesame 34, 36, 48, 150
Silicone 55, 60
Souccar 42
Spelt 36, 38, 48, 98, 124
Spielman 104
Spinach 39, 48
Sprout juice 68, 82, 116
Sprout-juice 58
St. John's wort 128, 152
Stanford University 44, 78, 140
Stepanoski 103
Strickgold 102
Sunflower 34, 35, 48, 60, 97, 147
Swansea University 38
Sweet potatoes 40

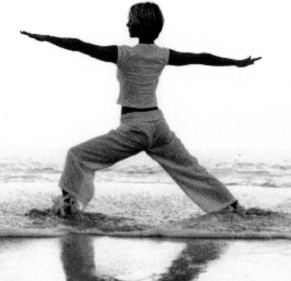

ValerieVHunt.com

Dépôt légal : novembre 2006
IMPRIMÉ EN FRANCE

Achevé d'imprimer le 10 novembre 2006
sur les presses de l'imprimerie «La Source d'Or»
63200 Marsat
Imprimeur n° 13580